THE
LEPTIN
BOOST
DIET

D0446075

THE LEPTIN BOOST DIET

Unleash Your Fat-Controlling
Hormones for Maximum Weight Loss

Scott Isaacs, M.D.

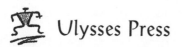 Ulysses Press

Text Copyright © 2007 Scott Isaacs. Design and Concept Copyright © 2007 Ulysses Press and its licensors. All rights reserved under International and Pan-American Copyright Conventions, including the right to reproduce this book or portions thereof in any form whatsoever, except for use by a reviewer in connection with a review.

Published by: Ulysses Press
P.O. Box 3440
Berkeley, CA 94703
www.ulyssespress.com

ISBN10: 1-56975-586-8
ISBN13: 978-1-56975-586-0
Library of Congress Control Number: 2006907932

Printed in Canada by Transcontinental Printing

10 9 8 7 6 5 4 3 2 1

Acquisitions Editor: Nicholas Denton-Brown
Managing Editor: Claire Chun
Editor: Mark Woodworth
Editorial and production staff: Lily Chou, Lisa Kester, Matt Orendorff, Elyce Petker
Index: Sayre Van Young
Cover design: Double R Design
Illustration on page 46 by Lindsay Mack

Distributed by Publishers Group West

NOTE TO READERS
This book has been written and published strictly for informational and educational purposes only. It is not intended to serve as medical advice or to be any form of medical treatment. You should always consult with your physician before altering or changing any aspect of your medical treatment. Do not stop or change any prescription medications without the guidance and advice of your physician. Any use of the information in this book is made on the reader's good judgment and is the reader's sole responsibility. This book is not intended to diagnose or treat any medical condition and is not a substitute for a physician.

This book is dedicated to Dr. Doug Coleman,
whose vision and pioneering research forever changed
our view of hormones and obesity.

TABLE OF CONTENTS

ACKNOWLEDGMENTS

I thank all my patients, past and present, for the knowledge they have given me about the multiple faces of hormonal balance and imbalance, and the privilege of being involved in their care. I also thank the staff at Intelligent Health Center, Janet Baldwin, R. N., Jennifer Kotze, Melva Baker, R. N., M.S., F.N.P.B.C., Beth Larker, Andrea Floyd, Shundalyn Vanderhorst, Deborah English, Luciana Neto, Rebecca Coelho M.S., R.D., L.D., and Fran Ritter, R.N. And I thank all the nurses in the diabetes units at Northside Hospital and Crawford Long Hospital for taking care of all my patients.

An extra special thanks goes to Jon Neihaus of Health Management Resources (HMR), whose insights and inspirations have helped our staff help our patients lose (and keep off) thousands of pounds. Thanks to Dean Felder, my trainer, who has kept me motivated to get in my PA (physical activity) so early in the morning. Thanks to Kalina Haynes and Tiffany Cochran of WXIA in Atlanta. Thanks to Kat Carney from CNN Headline News. Thanks to Julie Bitton, Tara Levine, and Mia Butler from TBS's "Movie and a Makeover." Thanks to Allison Winn Scotch and Hallie Levine for the interviews and including my opinions in their articles in *Men's Health, Women's Health, Prevention,* and other magazines. Thanks to Celia Rocks, Robyn Spizman, and Willy Spizman. I thank Lauren Handy of the American Association of Clinical Endocrinologists. And I thank my friends and colleagues Shaun Corbin, M.D., Randy Cleveland, M.D., David Shore, M.D., Karla Shore, M.D., Tom Flood,

M.D., Victor Silverman, M.D., Spencer Welch, M.D., Victoria Musey, M.D., David Arkin, M.D., Ola Odugbesan, M.D., Lewis Blevins, M.D., David Robertson, M.D., Tony Karpas, M.D., Kate Wheeler, M.D., Jim Christy, M.D., Chip Reed, M.D., Sabrina Rene, M.D., Jason Berner, M.D., Neil Shulman, M.D., Jason Holbrook, M.D., Todd Miller, M.D., Alan Miller, M.D., Dennis Steed, M.D., Judson Black, M.D., Joshua Barzilay, M.D., Guillermo Umpierrez, M.D., Bruce Trippe, M.D., Lee Padove, M.D., Andrew Golde, M.D., Kelly Ahn, M.D., Akin Ayodeji, M.D., Len Thaler, M.D., Jonathon Weinstein, M.D., Lee Oberman, M.D., Mitchell Blass, M.D., and Robyn Levy, M.D.

I thank my family and friends Howard Isaacs, Sheryle Isaacs, Steve Isaacs, Beverly Isaacs, Dick Isaacs, Marilyn Isaacs, Andy Rothberg, Sue Rothberg, Lorin Rothberg, Go Nodar, Manny Nodar, Bobbie Christmas, Jack Teitelman, Larry Teitelman, David Teitelman, Suzi Teitelman, Barbara Teitelman, Margaret Farrelly, Aaron Farrelly, Joyce Young, Brianna Young, John Little, IV, John Little, Sr., Stephen Gargan, Brenda Gargan, Rebecca Gargan, Laura Gargan, Jon Gunderson, Valerie Gunderson, Mark Luecke, Cynthia Cook, Travis Cook, Lori Johns, and Chase Johns.

Finally, I especially thank my wife, Fiona, who has put up with my working on the book at nights and on weekends and has given me the love and inspiration I needed to make this book into a reality.

Scott Isaacs, M.D.
Atlanta, Georgia

FOREWORD

Boosting Leptin

The key to achieving and maintaining a healthy body weight forever is to boost your leptin. Boosting leptin leads to a lifetime of good health. Boosting leptin is all about hormonal balance.

But what is *hormonal balance?*

Hormonal balance is a fairly vague term. In the world of health, though, it's like the Holy Grail. If you ask a gynecologist, he'll tell you it's the female hormones—estrogen and progesterone. If you ask a urologist, she'll tell you it's all about testosterone. If you ask diabetes experts, they'll tell you it's about balancing food and insulin. I take a different approach, for I believe that hormonal balance is about having *all* your hormones balanced. This is because all your hormones affect one another. It's one big circle, in a manner of speaking. When one hormone is out of whack, it produces profound effects on other hormones, which in turn change others. They are all connected. Hormonal balance means having the perfect amount of each and every hormone. It means having a body that's both healthy and resilient.

Hormones are your body's chemical messengers. They are the way your body communicates with itself. Being hormonally balanced means that you have gotten your body's communication system back on track. Good communication simply means having a healthy metabolism. If you are overweight or out of shape, that, in turn, means that your body has a communication problem.

Achieving hormonal balance by boosting leptin, adiponectin, and other fat cell hormones improves just about every aspect of your life. Your body will be lean and efficient. You won't feel excessive hunger or cravings, and your metabolism will work to keep your body at a healthy weight. You will feel more energetic, but without stress or anxiety. Your mood will be elevated. You will have deep, restful, rejuvenating sleep every night. You will have a sharp mind. Hormonal balance means feeling better and living longer.

As you read this book, you'll see how leptin, adiponectin, and other fat cell hormones are a vital part of hormonal balance. Problems with these hormones cause hormonal *im*balance, resulting in increased appetite, slower metabolism, and fat deposited in harmful areas like the belly and inside your muscles and organs. Balancing these fat cell hormones is critical for the proper functioning of your entire body.

Fat cell hormones are the hormonal link between your body and your brain. Of course, these hormones are affected by all your hormones and they, in turn, affect each other. When your fat cell hormones are balanced, all your hormones are balanced and your body can function at its best. And leptin is the key to fat cell hormonal balance.

When the body becomes obese, leptin doesn't work very well. That's called leptin resistance. You can give leptin a boost in two ways—by increasing production of leptin and by improving the way leptin works in the body. The Leptin Boost Diet is designed with both in mind. This book will teach you how to *boost* leptin by improving leptin resistance and enhancing leptin production. This will help you achieve hormonal balance *and* a healthy weight.

INTRODUCTION

The discovery of leptin in 1994 was one of the more significant breakthroughs in the history of obesity research. The name leptin comes from the Greek word *leptos,* which means "thin." Leptin is a hormone made by fat cells that tells your body to stop eating. The fat cells in your body work together to function like a gland, just like the adrenal gland, thyroid gland, or pituitary gland. Leptin works in your brain to control your appetite and metabolism. Leptin has led to the understanding that fat cells, also called *adipocytes,* are dynamic cells that produce hormones responsible for body weight, energy balance, metabolism, appetite, and food cravings.

In the past, scientists viewed fat as simply tissue that stores excess calories in the body. When obesity research began to be conducted, fat was thought of as an innocent bystander. But leptin has shattered our earlier perceptions of the fat cell. Scientists now understand that fat is much more than just an inert storage depot. Fat is a dynamic endocrine machine that is the critical regulator of your appetite, metabolism, and body weight.

Fat makes leptin. Leptin is the chemical messenger that allows your fat cells to communicate with your brain. Leptin tells the brain how much fat is in your body. As a person gains weight, leptin levels increase, extinguishing appetite and accelerating metabolism. Or that's how it's supposed to work. It turns out that leptin is pretty good at telling the brain that the body has *enough* fat, but leptin isn't as good at telling the brain that the body has *too much* fat. This is because as you gain weight, you develop *leptin resistance*. That's when the brain becomes blind to some of leptin's beneficial effects. Metabolism slows and you feel hungry even if you are overweight. If you want to lose weight and keep it off permanently, leptin must be able to work properly in your body. This means your fat cells must be able to make enough leptin, and your brain must be able to respond to it appropriately.

Since 1994, our knowledge of leptin has grown remarkably. In the first three years after its discovery, more than 800 scientific papers on leptin were published. Every obesity researcher seemed to be starting a "leptin lab." Today, global scientific meetings are held for researchers to share knowledge and ideas about leptin. Medical textbooks have been rewritten. New drugs are constantly being developed.

So it turns out that fat is not as boring as we once thought, and we have to rethink all our attitudes toward it.

PART I

THE FAT CELL IS AN ENDOCRINE ORGAN

1

LEPTIN, YOUR WEIGHT, AND YOUR HEALTH

Fat Is the Largest Gland in Your Body

Since the discovery of leptin, many more fat cell hormones have been discovered. All hormones made by fat cells affect your appetite, metabolism, and body weight. It's the body's form of self-regulation. Hormones made by fat are called *adipostatic* (*adipo* = fat, *static* = to stop) hormones because they regulate the amount of fat in the body. Leptin doesn't work alone. Adiponectin, resistin, visfatin, apelin, tumor necrosis factor-alpha, and interleukin-6 are only a few of the growing number of fat cell hormones that have been identified. Fat cells don't simply make hormones; they have receptors for hormones as well. Fat cells are regulated, in part, by traditional hormones like cortisol, insulin, and thyroid hormone. Traditional hormones work in concert with leptin to regulate your appetite, metabolism, and body weight. Many pharmaceutical companies have identified fat cell hormones as targets for new weight-loss medications; over two dozen are currently in development. As you read this book, the science of fat cell endocrinology is only in its infancy. Exciting discoveries surely lie ahead.

Endocrinology 101: Glands, Hormones, and Receptors

Hormones Are Chemical Messengers

To understand leptin, it's important to get a grasp of basic endocrinology—the science of glands and hormones. Most people I encounter in my practice or socially have never met an endocrinologist. They ask me, "What's an endocrinologist?" My answer is that an endocrinologist is a physician who specializes in glands and hormones. Endocrinology is a subspecialty of internal medicine that involves managing health problems that arise from hormone problems. Endocrinologists must complete four years of medical school, then five or six years of residency and fellowship training after medical school. The most common medical conditions treated by endocrinologists are diabetes, Polycystic Ovary Syndrome (PCOS), thyroid problems, pituitary gland problems, and male and female hormone problems. But endocrinologists manage hormone problems that affect just about every part of the body. Glands and tissues both produce hormones that deeply influence every known biological function. Anything you might imagine can go wrong—too much or too little hormone, hormone resistance, tumors and nodules in glands. When one hormone goes out of balance, others follow.

The endocrine system is your body's system of communication. Hormonal balance means good communication. Hormones are chemical messengers produced by glands and other tissues and are secreted into the bloodstream where they cause actions at a distant location in the body. Different types of hormones produce different effects. Some hormones are made from cholesterol, while others are made from protein. Even though leptin and adiponectin are made by fat cells, they are protein hormones. Hormones are responsible for how your body communicates with its various organs and systems to control all their functions. All living organisms have hormones.

Traditional hormones come from distinct glands, such as the thyroid gland, adrenal gland, ovaries, and testicles. These hormones are controlled by the pituitary gland, also known as the *master gland*. The pituitary gland is regulated by other parts of the brain, including the *hypothalamus*. All your hormones influence one another. Your body contains an elegant yet delicate system to keep your hormones in balance.

Modern discoveries have taught us that every organ or tissue in the body can act like a gland, with the ability to make hormones. Fat cells, for instance, make hormones. And so do nerves, the stomach and intestines, the liver, even the heart and kidneys. A single cell has the capability to produce many different types of hormones. Hormones travel through the bloodstream, bringing their signals to various parts of the body.

When a hormone finds its target, it binds with a specific receptor, like a key slipping into a lock. As a hormone and receptor merge, the door is unlocked and a chain of events begins. The action of a hormone depends on the location of the receptor. When thyroid hormone binds with its receptor on the heart, for example, the heart beats faster, and when the same thyroid hormone binds with its receptor on the intestines, they move faster as well.

Leptin receptors are found throughout the entire body, but their main location is the appetite control center, located in the brain. Leptin is the chemical messenger that transmits signals from fat cells directly to the brain. When leptin binds with the brain's receptors, it shuts down appetite and speeds up metabolism.

Hormonal Rhythms

We humans are intimately connected to the earth and its rotation, day and night, light and dark. We all have an internal biological clock that is linked to our hormones. Daily rhythms have a profound effect on our hormones and metabolism. Hormones are constantly changing. They are always going up or down. The natural hormonal ebb and flow has evolved over thousands of generations. We need different hormones to peak at different times of the day. Hormones that make blood sugar rise peak around dawn, to help our body get going in the morning. Other hormones, like growth hormone and leptin, surge in the middle of the night, while we're sleeping. Some hormones are produced in small bursts every few minutes, or every few hours. Some hormones even change with the seasons. Hormonal fluctuations throughout the day are a fundamental part of natural hormonal balance. Anything that disrupts our sleep-wake cycle will disrupt our diurnal rhythm, and our hormones will go out of balance. People with sleeping problems, overseas travelers, night-shift or swing-shift workers, all frequently have hormone problems because their diurnal rhythms are out of kilter.

DIURNAL RHYTHMS

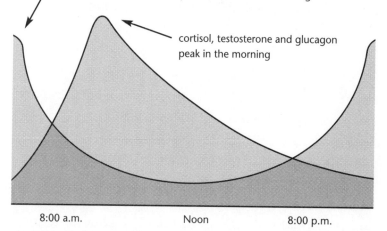

leptin and growth hormone peak in the middle of the night

cortisol, testosterone and glucagon peak in the morning

| 8:00 a.m. | Noon | 8:00 p.m. |

Hormone levels vary throughout the day. Leptin and growth hormone peak in the middle of the night. This is why eating in the middle of the night (between 2 a.m. and 4 a.m.) can disrupt hormonal balance and lead to weight gain. Cortisol, testosterone, and glucagon peak around 8 a.m. and are at their lowest point in the late afternoon.

Communication Problems

Hormone problems mean communication problems. If the body can't produce the proper amounts of hormones, the organs can't communicate with each other and things start to break down. Good communication, therefore, is vital to a healthy metabolism.

When a gland fails, hormonal deficiency occurs. That's what we see in conditions like hypothyroidism, which occurs when the thyroid gland stops making thyroid hormones, or menopause, when the ovaries stop making estrogen. Type 1 diabetes occurs when the

LEPTIN DEFICIENCY AND LEPTIN RESISTANCE

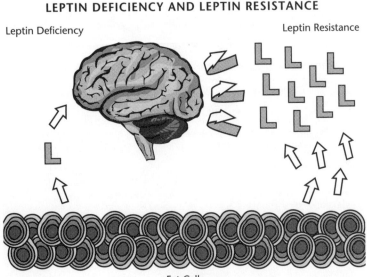

Leptin Deficiency

Leptin Resistance

Fat Cells

Leptin deficiency occurs when fat cells cannot produce the hormone leptin. Leptin resistance occurs when leptin cannot work properly. The body's natural response to hormone resistance is to produce excess hormone. On the surface, hormone deficiency and hormone resistance can appear the same. Leptin deficiency and leptin resistance both result in obesity, because the brain thinks the body is starving. In the early stages of leptin resistance, fat cells ramp up leptin production and can overcome the resistance. If you reach a point when you are no longer able to make enough leptin to keep up with the demand, this is called a "relative" leptin deficiency, even though leptin levels are high. If you are overweight, you have a combination of leptin resistance and a relative leptin deficiency. Treatments are focused on boosting leptin by increasing leptin production while alleviating leptin resistance. Leptin is indicated by the letter L.

pancreas stops making insulin. Leptin deficiency exists as well, and, just as you might expect, people with leptin deficiency are extremely obese. This is a very rare condition, however. Most people who are obese do *not* have leptin deficiency.

Glands can become overactive, resulting in hormonal excess. Cushing's syndrome is a condition in which the pituitary gland or the adrenal gland, or both, are overactive, resulting in too much cortisol. Excess cortisol stimulates appetite and increases fat storage in the body, causing massive weight gain. Hyperthyroidism occurs when the thyroid gland makes too much thyroid hormone. A tumor in the pancreas known as an insulinoma can produce very high insulin levels, causing weight gain and dangerously low blood sugar. Hormonal excess can be as devastating as hormonal deficiency. Treatments for hormonal excess include medications, radiation, or sometimes surgical removal of the offending gland.

Too much or too little of a particular hormone causes hormonal imbalance.

Sometimes the problem is not with the gland but with the receptor for a particular hormone. When a receptor becomes dysfunctional, this is known as *resistance*. In many ways, having hormone resistance is similar to having hormone deficiency. This is because hormone resistance makes the body blind to the effects of a hormone. Type 1 diabetes, for example, is caused by insulin deficiency, while type 2 diabetes is caused by insulin resistance. On the surface, the two diseases may appear identical, although one is caused by hormone deficiency and the other by hormone resistance. It's the same with leptin: people with leptin deficiency and those with leptin resistance are both overweight.

In states of hormone resistance, the hormone levels are high because the body is trying to compensate for faulty receptors. The body's natural response is to produce excess hormone to overcome the resistance. Hormonal excess is a hallmark of hormone resistance.

Weight gain causes many hormone receptors to malfunction. The insulin receptor is the one that everyone talks about. Insulin resistance is an unavoidable consequence of weight gain. But it turns out that leptin resistance is also a major problem caused by excess weight. Leptin resistance and insulin resistance almost always occur together. Most people who are overweight have very high levels of both insulin and leptin as their body tries to overcome the resistance. The best treatments for hormone resistance focus on improving the way a receptor functions—that is, alleviating the resistance. But sometimes doctors take the attitude of "if you can't beat 'em, join 'em" and treat hormone resistance by giving even more hormones. The classic example is end stage type 2 diabetes, when insulin injections are required to treat high blood sugar levels. This strategy was also tried by treating leptin resistance with injections of synthetic leptin. Unfortunately, the results from initial trials were disappointing. Ongoing research in this area continues, and perhaps one day leptin resistance will be treated by giving injections of leptin. I suspect, however, that we are more likely to find a solution from making the leptin receptor work better, instead of trying to overpower it with megadoses of synthetic leptin.

The truth is that most endocrine diseases are not so clear cut; they are more a combination of hormone imbalance and hormone resistance. Obesity, for example, is actually a combination of leptin resistance and leptin deficiency. This is because if you had enough leptin to overcome the resistance, there wouldn't be a problem. This is known as a "relative leptin deficiency." As you continue through this book, you'll see that most people can experience problems with leptin either from increasing leptin resistance or from decreasing leptin production. The treatments I'll discuss are focused on boosting leptin by improving leptin resistance while at the same time increasing leptin production.

For more information on your body's hormonal systems, please see my book *Hormonal Balance: Understanding Hormones, Weight, and Your Metabolism* (Bull Publishing, 2006, second edition).

Stress and Your Hormones

Stress causes hormonal imbalance in a great many ways. Stress causes leptin resistance, insulin resistance, lower sex hormones (estrogen in women, testosterone in men), lower levels of growth hormone, and higher cortisol levels. Stress also reduces the body's ability to convert thyroid hormone to an active form, thus reducing its efficiency. Each one of these hormonal changes slows metabolism and causes weight gain.

A dynamic relationship exists between the stress in your life, your hormones, and your brain. Stress can actually rewire parts of the brain, resulting in memory problems and depression. The brain's response to stress can make you feel anxious, tired, angry, frustrated, or hungry. You don't feel like exercising and are more likely to smoke or drink excessive alcohol when you are under stress.

You undoubtedly are familiar with various types of stress. You can have emotional stress, stress from life, stress from your job or your family. You can experience stress from a poor diet, lack of exercise, or poor general health, all of which can be equally damaging to hormonal balance. If you don't get enough sleep or enough good-

STRESS AND YOUR HORMONES

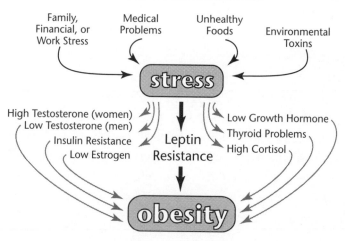

quality sleep, it will put tremendous stress on your endocrine system. Toxins from our environment, such as pesticides or traces of chemicals in food and drinking water, add stress to our systems. It's not just about being "stressed out" by other people or situations. Stress of *any* type causes hormonal imbalance, which leads to weight gain. But not all stress is bad. Short-term stress can be challenging and invigorating. The key to losing weight and keeping it off is minimizing the bad stress on your body.

Chronic Fatigue

In my practice as an endocrinologist, one of the more common complaints I hear from my patients is that they have poor energy levels. They describe the feeling as fatigue, low energy, tiredness, exhaustion, drowsiness, or all the above. Many patients describe waking up feeling as if their sleep was unrestful. Others tell me that they start the day feeling fine, but become totally exhausted by midafternoon. For some people, the tiredness occurs every day, while for others it comes intermittently. Some of my patients have been through extensive medical evaluations to check for the more common (and even not so common) causes of fatigue. They have been checked for sleep apnea, anemia, infection, immune system problems, heart problems, kidney problems, liver problems, and traditional hormonal problems like hypothyroidism and diabetes. Their evaluation keeps coming up normal. Some of these patients are told they have depression, chronic fatigue, or fibromyalgia.

It is always a challenge for doctors to determine the cause of patients' fatigue. Hundreds of causes could be contributing factors, and running a battery of tests that come back "normal" does not always mean that everything really *is* normal. In my experience, most people who are told they have "chronic fatigue syndrome" actually have a different underlying cause of the fatigue. The key is discovering the cause, then treating it.

Identifying the cause of someone's fatigue can be challenging—for everything must be investigated. A hidden infection (say, in the gums or the sinuses) may be the cause of chronic fatigue. Sometimes chronic fatigue is caused by deficiency of a particular nutrient or vitamin. Sometimes fatigue is caused by hormonal imbalance that is not severe enough to be detected by routine testing.

Fatigue is commonly caused by problems with leptin, adiponectin, or other fat cell hormones. These hormones are the regulators of your body's ability to burn nutrients or store nutrients—in short, your metabolism. They are the key to switching your body from fat storage mode to fat burning mode. When you are in fat storage mode, leptin and adiponectin are low. The food you eat is converted to fat and is deposited in the unhealthy regions of the body—in the belly and inside the muscles and organs. You feel tired all the time, because your body is converting the food you eat into fat instead of burning it as energy. Your muscles become flabby, and fat builds up inside your belly. The organs and blood vessels begin to fill with fat, eventually leading to more fatigue and serious health problems. If you shift your body into fat burning mode, the food you eat and the excess fat in your body will be converted energy, making you feel energetic. The Leptin Boost Diet will help you regain control of your hormones. You'll shift back into fat burning mode, and you'll experience a dramatic improvement in your energy level.

Many people who have been told they have "chronic fatigue syndrome" are in fact tired because they have an imbalance of fat cell hormones, brain hormones, gut hormones, or other hormones. As you read the pages of this book, I'll talk about many of your hormones and how problems with them will affect leptin, adiponectin, and others, causing fatigue. By balancing your fat cell hormones, you can achieve a total hormonal balance that will help you regain your energy and feel good all the time.

Diabesity

The term *diabesity* has been used to describe the intimate link between diabetes and obesity. They're connected in a critical way. Leptin and adiponectin are key hormones responsible for this link. In the past 25 years the number of people diagnosed with diabetes has increased considerably. It has doubled in only the last 10 years. According to the National Institute of Diabetes and Digestive and Kidney Disease (NIDDK), more than 20 million adults over the age of 20 in the United States have type 2 diabetes. And 55 million adults have more-subtle blood sugar abnormalities known as *prediabetes*. In total, 35 percent of the U.S. adult population—about 105 million people—has diabetes or prediabetes. Some 90 percent of people with newly diagnosed diabetes are overweight. The increase in diabetes rates parallels the rapid increase in obesity rates seen over the past three decades.

The *Metabolic Syndrome* is a newly described condition that includes diabetes or prediabetes, increased fat in the belly, high blood pressure, high triglycerides, and low good (HDL) cholesterol. The established criteria to diagnose Metabolic Syndrome are what most physicians would consider "high normal." You only have to have three of the five criteria to qualify for Metabolic Syndrome. This makes it extremely common—55 million Americans have it. Although insulin resistance has been thought of as the driving force behind Metabolic Syndrome, experts agree that it's much more complicated than that. A multitude of hormones are out of balance; leptin and adiponectin are on the top of the list. Insulin resistance, leptin resistance, and low adiponectin levels go hand in hand.

Metabolic Syndrome is a major risk factor for cardiovascular disease—or heart attacks and strokes. This has led to the trend for doctors to aggressively treat all the components of the syndrome. It's now considered the "medical standard of care" to use medications to treat conditions that typically produce no symptoms. This means using medications both to treat insulin resistance and to treat mildly elevated blood pressure or slightly high blood fats. By doing so, and by treating the problems early and aggressively, doctors hope that their patients can avoid more severe complications. For more detailed information on Metabolic Syndrome, its causes, and its treatments, please read my book *Overcoming Metabolic Syndrome* (Addicus Books, 2005).

Preventing Cardiovascular Disease

Being overweight significantly increases your risk for developing many medical problems, but the No. 1 cause of death in obese people is cardiovascular disease. By the time most people develop symptoms, their cardiovascular disease is already at an advanced stage. As soon as you start to gain weight, your hormones and metabolism begin to change. Leptin, along with other hormones like insulin, becomes dysfunctional. The body becomes resistant to the effects of hormones, resulting in hormonal imbalance.

At first, you won't find any symptoms from hormone resistance, or your symptoms will be so subtle that you can easily overlook them: fatigue, feeling bloated or tired after dinner, carbohydrate cravings, getting tired walking up a flight of stairs, dizziness, frequent urination, or slightly blurred vision. As time goes on, your problems usually intensify and magnify each other. Blood sugar, blood pressure, and blood fats (cholesterol and triglycerides) all go up. Eventually, these metabolic derangements damage your cardiovascular system.

Of course, it's never too late to reverse this cycle. But the good news is that the earlier you break it, the lower your risk of dying from cardiovascular disease. As a physician, I've seen the trend— the huge push toward preventative medicine. It's a wonderful example of how years of research have produced results and medications that are being brought back to real people to help improve their lives. We doctors are more compulsive than ever about screening and monitoring our patients for the conditions that are treatable, and we often can prevent cardiovascular disease or even reverse it in those who already have it. And we're treating these problems more and more aggressively. What once may have been considered "high normal" is now overtly high in many cases. More and more medications are being developed to treat high blood sugar, high blood fats, and high blood pressure because we know that treating these problems reduces the risk of our patients' cardiovascular disease and death.

The problem is: where do we stop? I've seen patients start on one medication for blood pressure and within 5 years they are on 10 different medications! In fact, most people these days need "combination drug therapy" to treat their blood pressure, blood sugar, cholesterol, and triglycerides. Often we forget that simply balancing our hormones and losing weight will cure these ailments, eliminating the need for drugs altogether. It's all about balance. I strongly support the use of medications and, as a physician, I prescribe them every day. There's plenty of science to show that some of these medications truly are medical breakthroughs. But I also discontinue medications or reduce the dose in my patients who have achieved hormonal balance and have lost weight. My approach is to prescribe medications for my patients that will treat the immediate medical problems but will also help balance their hormones to allow their bodies to function more efficiently. It's never perfect, but many medications that have the primary goal of treating diabetes, high blood pressure, high cholesterol, or other conditions can have the extra benefit of improving hormonal balance as well. Yet other medications can *cause* hormonal imbalance, appearing to improve a condition while in fact only covering it up. As you read this book, you'll learn about many of the medications that I prescribe in my medical endocrinology practice and how they affect leptin, adiponectin, and the rest of your hormones.

Endothelial Dysfunction:
The Ticking Time Bomb

Cardiovascular disease is the leading cause of death in the United States. The modern scientific view of the cardiovascular (*cardio* = heart, *vascular* = blood vessels) system is very similar to our new view of the fat cell. Just as we used to think of fat as a depot to store excess calories, we once viewed the cardiovascular system as merely a system of pipes. We now know that the cardiovascular system is a

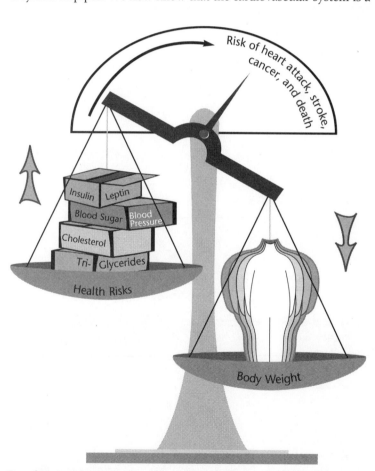

Everything is going UP! As you gain weight, risk increases. Weight loss lowers your risk for a host of medical problems and helps you achieve hormonal balance.

sophisticated network of arteries, veins, and capillaries made up of highly specialized cells. The inner lining, known as the *endothelium*, is a fragile layer of dynamic cells that are the key regulators of cardiovascular health. Cardiovascular disease, then, is the result of injury or damage to the endothelium. Constantly bathed by passing blood, *endothelial cells* are influenced by everything about the blood—blood sugar, blood pressure, blood fats, and hormones. The endothelial cell is extremely fragile and easily injured. *Endothelial dysfunction* is the earliest form of cardiovascular disease. With time, endothelial

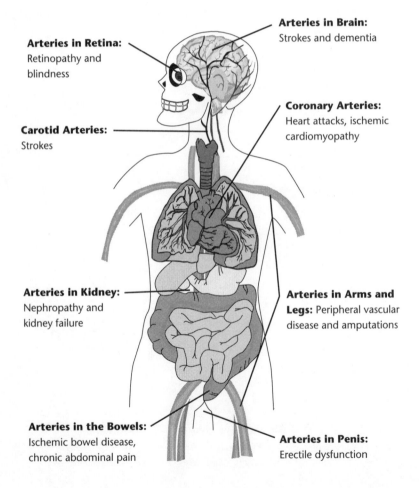

Arteries in Brain: Strokes and dementia

Arteries in Retina: Retinopathy and blindness

Coronary Arteries: Heart attacks, ischemic cardiomyopathy

Carotid Arteries: Strokes

Arteries in Kidney: Nephropathy and kidney failure

Arteries in Arms and Legs: Peripheral vascular disease and amputations

Arteries in the Bowels: Ischemic bowel disease, chronic abdominal pain

Arteries in Penis: Erectile dysfunction

dysfunction progresses to atherosclerosis, or hardening of the arteries. This is the fundamental cause of cardiovascular disease.

Every part of the body is linked to the cardiovascular system and depends on it for its very existence. And that's why there are so many different types of problems associated with cardiovascular disease. Disease of the coronary arteries can lead to coronary heart disease (CHD) or to a heart attack. Disease of the carotid arteries or arteries in the brain can cause a stroke or dementia. Problems with the blood vessels in the arms or legs can cause peripheral vascular disease (PVD), which is a leading cause of amputations. Diseases of other blood vessels can cause kidney disease, blindness, nerve damage, bowel problems, even erectile dysfunction.

So instead of looking at the cardiovascular system as just a set of pipes, think about the delicate endothelial cells lining those pipes. If the lining is healthy, your cardiovascular system is healthy. But wherever that delicate lining gets damaged, the organ that it's connected to pays the price. The endothelial cells function as a unit. If there are signs of damage in one area, you can almost be sure that your entire cardiovascular system is diseased. It's just a matter of time before you'll develop problems in other areas as well.

The Tip of the Iceberg

While cardiovascular disease is the most common complication to being overweight, it's not the only one. The list of medical complications linked to excess weight seems, unfortunately, to be getting longer and longer. There's a cascade of problems, all of which begin with leptin. When leptin is out of balance, the whole body gets out of balance. The heavier you are, the more likely you are to have a problem with fat cell hormones, and the greater your risk of having medical problems. After all, weight loss is about more than just looking better. It's about being healthier, feeling better, and living longer.

MEDICAL PROBLEMS LINKED TO OBESITY	
Acne	Hirsutism
Amputations	Hypertension
Anxiety	Infertility
Arthritis	Insomnia
Asthma	Kidney disease
Back pain	Low testosterone, in men
Cancer (all types)	Male breast growth
Cardiomyopathy	Metabolic Syndrome
Cardiovascular disease	Osteoarthritis
Charcot joints	Peripheral Vascular Disease
Chronic Fatigue Syndrome	Polycystic Ovary Syndrome
Chronic pain	Poor wound healing
Depression	Prediabetes
Diabetes	Premature death
Diverticulosis	Pseudocushing's Syndrome
Edema	Pulmonary hypertension
Fatigue	Restrictive lung disease
Foot ulcers	Skin problems
Gallstones	Sleep apnea
Gastroesophageal Reflux Disease	Strokes
Gout	Swelling
Heart attacks	Varicose veins
High testosterone, in women	Venous Stasis Disease

The best way to lose weight and keep it off permanently is through hormonal balance. Leptin is critical in this process. As you read this book, you will learn how to overcome leptin resistance so that you can lose weight effortlessly and permanently without hunger or cravings. You will be healthier and will lower your risk of a multitude of ailments.

2

FAT CELL HORMONES

Early Leptin Research

Oddly enough, the lowly mouse has been one of the more powerful tools in the history of obesity research. Many human diseases have been mimicked in mice, making this common animal an ideal platform for research. Obese mice have been a major target of obesity research for many decades.

In 1902, a French scientist named L. Cuenot described an obese yellow mouse that had been bred by European mouse fanciers since the 1800s. This was the first-ever report of a naturally obese mouse. This led to the investigation of other obese mice, including the leptin-deficient *obese* mouse. The obese yellow mouse led to the subsequent discovery of melanocortin, a brain hormone that's ultimately linked to leptin.

In the late 1940s, a mutant strain of mice was found to have a syndrome of obesity and related complications quite similar to what we now call Metabolic Syndrome in humans. These mice seemed hungry all the time and had high insulin levels, increased body fat, high cortisol levels, low thyroid levels, and high blood sugar. In addition, they had a low body temperature, indicating low metabolism. The mice were infertile and showed low levels of estrogen and testosterone. Scientists believed that this *obese* mouse (called an *ob*) lacked a *satiety factor*—a hormone, still undiscovered, that they called "leptin."

In the 1970s, a scientist named Doug Coleman preformed a series of classic experiments to prove that theory. These studies, known as *parabiosis experiments*, sought to establish leptin's existence. Parabiosis is not the type of experiment that is performed on humans. Two mice are joined surgically, right down to their circulation, like artificial Siamese twins. Hormones made in one mouse, therefore, are transferred to the other mouse.

When an *ob* mouse was joined with a normal mouse, an amazing thing occurred. The obese mouse lost weight! The theory was strengthened: these obese mice lacked a hormone that shut off appetite in the brain.

The *ob/ob* mouse is the scientific term for Coleman's obese mouse, which is now known to be a mouse with severe leptin deficiency. The *ob/ob* mouse has very particular characteristics. It's a fat mouse, three or four times the weight of a normal mouse, and it keeps eating. The *ob/ob* mouse is hungry all the time. Scientists have found that the *ob/ob* mouse has a mutated leptin gene. There are actually two copies of each leptin gene, and *ob/ob* indicates that both leptin genes (also know as the *ob* gene) are defective. The *ob/ob* mouse is used as a research model for studying leptin deficiency. It has slow metabolism and low body temperature as well as severe, early-onset type 2 diabetes as well as infertility. It has high cortisol, low testosterone, and low thyroid hormone levels.

Coleman also performed experiments on a second strain of mice known as the *db* mouse (named for its propensity for diabetes). The *db* mouse was also obese, and on the surface appeared to be very similar to an *ob* mouse. He found that when he joined the circulation of the *db* mouse with that of a normal mouse, the normal mouse died of starvation. Colman inferred that the *db* mouse had very high leptin levels due to a mutated receptor for leptin—in other words, leptin resistance. His theories have since been confirmed by other scientific research.

Research Breakthrough: Finding the Leptin Gene

Dr. Coleman hypothesized that the *ob* mouse had leptin deficiency and the *db* mouse had leptin resistance. In the 1980s, obesity researchers Spiegelman and Flier proved for the first time that fat cells

COLEMAN'S PARABIOSIS MICE

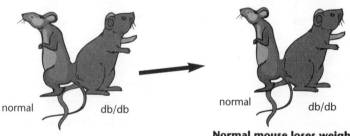

normal ob/ob → normal ob/ob

Obese mouse loses weight

Experiment #1

Fat Mouse (ob/ob) Next to Normal Mouse (normal) Becomes 2 Normal Mice

When leptin is transferred from the normal mouse to the leptin-deficient mouse (obese) mouse, it loses weight.

normal db/db → normal db/db

Normal mouse loses weight

Experiment #2

Fat Mouse (db/db) Next to Normal Mouse (normal) Becomes Fat Mouse and Very Skinny Mouse

When excess leptin is transferred from the leptin-resistant mouse (db/db) to the normal mouse, it causes the normal mouse to stop eating and the mouse becomes malnourished.

produced a protein, called *adipsin* or *complement factor D*. But it wasn't until 1994 that Jeffrey Friedman and colleagues cloned the gene for leptin (known as the *ob* gene) and Coleman's theory was confirmed. Genes are responsible for making a specific protein, and when it comes to the *ob* gene, its protein product (once called the *ob* protein) is leptin. The *ob* gene is the leptin gene. The *ob* receptor is the leptin receptor.

Around the same time, other scientists described a protein that was initially termed Acrp30, which later became known as *adiponectin*. Adiponectin and leptin were the first of many fat cell hormones yet to be discovered. I'll talk more about these hormones later in this chapter.

Once the leptin protein was identified, scientists quickly figured out how to measure it in the blood stream. They found that the *ob* mouse had very low leptin levels. The *db* mouse had very high leptin levels. They had two obese mice, one with low and the other with high leptin levels. The *ob* mouse had a defective gene for leptin, causing *leptin deficiency*. The *db* mouse had a defective gene for the leptin receptor, causing *leptin resistance*.

Researchers easily learned how to create genetically engineered leptin, known as *recombinant leptin*. The process used to make leptin today is similar to that used to make insulin and other hormonal medications.

Recombinant leptin was given to the *ob* mouse. It then showed decreased food intake, increased metabolism, and dramatic weight loss. Within weeks, the mouse appeared normal. Eventually, humans with leptin deficiency were located in a family in Pakistan and the first human research trials began. Leptin injections caused dramatic weight loss in these individuals—without diet or exercise!

One year after the discovery of leptin, the leptin receptor was identified. It didn't take long because researchers knew where to look—the hunger centers of the brain. They knew to look for a receptor for leptin, because all hormones have receptors. It was only logical to start where leptin was hypothesized to work.

While they initially focused on the effects of leptin in the brain, other researchers discovered important actions in other tissues too. Leptin plays a role in directly regulating immune cells, reproductive cells, pancreatic cells, bone cells, fat cells, muscle cells, and even cancer cells. Leptin regulates the inner workings of muscles, thereby affecting insulin sensitivity and blood sugar. Recent progress in understanding the way the leptin receptor works has uncovered potential new targets for drug research in obesity and diabetes.

Following the discovery of leptin and its receptor, the scientific and medical communities have expressed hope that leptin-like medications will lead to a cure for obesity. Leptin injections were investigated as a treatment for obese humans with leptin resistance, although the results were disappointing. It is thought that leptin had trouble penetrating what's known as the *blood-brain barrier*. Today, leptin injections are only a miracle and medical breakthrough for people with leptin deficiency, a very rare condition. Research is currently underway, investigating leptin as a way of helping people who have lost weight to keep it off.

We are learning that the role of leptin is more complex than we ever imagined. Scientists now understand that leptin interacts with many hormones in the brain and throughout the body. Leptin has a variety of roles that go far beyond appetite, metabolism, and body weight. It acts as a growth factor, as a regulator of puberty and fertility, as an immune system regulator, and as a modulator of the fetus with the maternal metabolism. Most importantly in all these interactions, it also interacts with other hormones, like insulin, glucagon, growth hormone, thyroid hormone, testosterone, estrogen, and cortisol. Recently, leptin has also been found to be an important factor responsible for the growth of blood vessels and bones in a developing fetus as well as in cancerous tumors.

Leptin Deficiency Versus Leptin Resistance

In many ways, leptin deficiency and leptin resistance are alike. Understanding the hormone insulin and how it leads to diabetes is helpful in understanding the differences and similarities between leptin deficiency and leptin resistance. Both insulin deficiency and resistance cause diabetes. But many people with diabetes appear the same on the outside, even though the underlying cause of the diabetes may be quite different. Type 1 diabetes is a relatively uncommon form of diabetes, and is also known as juvenile onset diabetes or insulin dependent diabetes mellitus (IDDM). The hallmark of type 1 diabetes is insulin deficiency caused by immune system destruction of insulin-producing cells in the pancreas. Type 2 diabetes is a more common form of diabetes, associated with obesity and insulin resistance.

As with most things in life, though, it's not really that simple. For example, many overweight people with type 1 diabetes have underlying insulin resistance, what endocrinologists refer to as "double diabetes." And experts say that people with type 2 diabetes have, in reality, a combination of insulin resistance and insulin deficiency. This is because even though their body is making huge amounts of insulin, it is not enough to keep blood sugars in the normal range. This is known as a "relative deficiency," but with time the pancreas gets "burned out" and it makes less and less insulin. Either way— whether an insulin deficiency, a resistance, or a combination of the two—the end result is the same: diabetes.

The same situation exists with leptin. Leptin deficiency, like type 1 diabetes, is a rare condition. But leptin resistance, like type 2 diabetes, is common. Both leptin deficiency and resistance appear the same from the outside: as obesity. And as with diabetes, leptin problems rarely occur in isolation, since most sufferers have a combination of both leptin resistance and deficiency—leaning more heavily on the resistance side. This is important when applying scientific research to the real world. Most research focuses on either leptin deficiency or leptin resistance, not a combination. In fact, many assumptions that we make about leptin resistance are based on research that focused on leptin deficiency, or vice versa. At its root, boosting leptin means alleviating leptin deficiency and improving leptin resistance at the same time.

Leptin's Importance during Prehistoric Times

Leptin has been vital for survival throughout the generations, for it prevented humans from dying of starvation. That is its true role—to prevent the body from perishing from lack of food . Until very recently, starvation had been the major cause of death for human beings. Dean Ornish has wittily said that thousands of years ago "it was survival of the fattest."

Our hormonal systems have developed with the goal of preventing malnutrition. In the grand timeline of human existence, it's been just a millisecond since food became as plentiful as it is today in developed countries. Yet our hormones haven't had time to catch up. Since leptin's role is to function as a communicator of the body's nutritional status, it signals the brain, letting it know whether the body is starving or that everything is OK. If fat stores are low and starvation is a risk, a body's leptin levels will be low, increasing hunger and slowing metabolism.

Leptin has not fared well, however, in our modern epidemic of obesity, because it's not accustomed to dealing with too much fat. It was always intended to prevent the body's having too *little* fat. So, when the body becomes overweight, leptin doesn't work quite right. Leptin doesn't protect us from obesity the way it protects us from starvation. But you can still lose weight through leptin. Follow the lessons in this book and you'll be on your way to a healthy leptin system and overall hormonal balance.

The Appetite Control System

Is it possible to control your appetite? First, you'll want to know about the huge number of chemical signals that influence our appetite, metabolism, and body weight. These hormonal signals unlock the secret of the most important health problem of our generation. The science in this area is advancing at a dizzying pace. Leptin is indeed a powerful hormonal regulator of appetite. But many hormones regulate our *appetite control system,* and if any one goes out of balance, it's likely that others will also fall, like dominoes.

The appetite control system contains five basic parts. Each part, a different system of hormones, influences the others. It's the most intricate system of communication in our body. Dozens, if not hundreds, of hormones are dancing around in your body. Each one has a slightly different effect on appetite, hunger, satiety (or feeling full), and cravings. Leptin, for example, has its most potent influence on long-term body weight, how satisfied you feel after a meal, and the amount of fat in your body. Leptin has a lesser effect on your appetite and cravings from one moment to the next. This is more the realm of hormones like insulin and hormones made by your digestive system. But it's never 100 percent. These hunger hormones all have some effect on your daily appetite and cravings, as well as your body weight over the long term and your overall metabolism.

The *set point* is the brain's opinion of how much you should weigh. This internal drive is universal for all animals, including humans. The brain has powerful subconscious influences over feeding behaviors, such as satiety, hunger and cravings, metabolism, and energy level. The brain's internal feeding drives are very powerful indeed. These drives can easily overcome "willpower" as you try to lose weight. The set point is an adaptive response to protect the body from starvation. It's all about survival. If the brain senses that the body is starving, it will work to reverse this condition.

But how can the brain sense whether you are malnourished or, in fact, overweight? Through leptin. Leptin tells the brain exactly

THE APPETITE CONTROL SYSTEM

Nervous System: Hunger centers in the hypothalamus as well as in other areas of the brain are responsive to leptin, adiponectin, insulin, thyroid hormone, and many others. The brain, spinal cord, and nerves make hormones that oversee the appetite control system, regulate fat cells, control metabolism, and affect the digestive system. The brain has influence over the production of many hormones through the pituitary gland. Potent nervous system hunger hormones include neuropeptide Y, POMC, dopamine, serotonin, GABA, galanin, and many others.

Metabolic Hormones: Insulin, thyroid hormone, growth hormone, testosterone, estrogen, and many other hormones and molecules influence the appetite control system. Hormones coordinate to regulate all aspects of appetite and satiety.

Fat Cell Hormones: Leptin, adiponectin, visfatin, resistin, and other fat cell hormones communicate with the body to self-regulate size and number. They have a strong influence on appetite as it contributes to overall weight.

Gut Hormones: Ghrelin, incretins (GLP-1 & GIP), cholecystokinin, glucagon, and other hormones produced by the digestive system affect the appetite on a moment's notice and are strongly affected by food.

Inflammatory Cytokines: TNF-α, IL-6, and other toxic substances are produced by the body as part of inflammation. Fat cells make cytokines, known as adipokines, which decrease appetite and are blamed for weight loss seen in cancer victims. In overweight people, the appetite-suppressing effect of TNF-α and IL-6 is overwhelmed by their ability to cause leptin and insulin resistance as well as other hormonal problems, so their overall effect is bad. Interestingly, the structure of leptin is similar to that of other cytokine hormones.

how much fat is in your body. Under normal circumstances, the more fat you have, the more leptin is produced. When leptin levels are low, you feel hungry. When leptin is high, you feel less hungry, and when you do eat, the meal is more satisfying. If the brain does not get enough leptin, it believes the body is malnourished (even if you are overweight) and sets in motion a hormonal cascade that stimulates feeding behaviors and slows metabolism. This is a protective mechanism. It is to protect you from starvation.

If you don't have enough leptin, or your leptin doesn't work properly, the brain thinks the body is starving—even if the reality is to the contrary. This communication problem disrupts normal hormonal balance. The brain's main concern is survival—since we are genetically hardwired to survive famines. Today's environment of high-calorie foods goes against our evolutionary instincts. "Becoming obese," says obesity expert Dr. James Hill of the University of Colorado, "is a normal response to the American environment."

The brain has not evolved as quickly as our society's ability to make food readily available at virtually all times and places. And although the food environment has completely evolved in ways that would astonish our ancestors, human brains today are not much different than our ancestors'. "Genetics loads the gun. Environment pulls the trigger," says obesity expert Dr. George Bray.

As you gain weight, more leptin is produced because there's more hormone-producing fat. But somehow the wires get crossed. The brain becomes "resistant" to leptin's effects. Leptin resistance means the brain becomes "blind" to leptin. Even when leptin levels are high, that leptin is invisible to the brain. In confusion, the brain thinks the body's starving, even though it's overweight. It keeps sending out signals to gain weight, eat more, not starve. To be effective in losing weight, therefore, you have to satisfy your brain's need for leptin.

You have to uncross the wires—alleviate leptin resistance and open your brain's "eyes," so that it can see the reality of your weight. Once the brain can recognize your true body weight, your appetite will be dramatically reduced and cravings will be eliminated, metabolism will speed up, energy expenditure will increase, and weight loss will become much easier as your brain works with you, instead of against you.

Leptin is the reason why many diets fail. If your leptin is not balanced, your brain will work against you as you try to lose weight. But you can harness the power of leptin to tell your subconscious brain to work with you, not against you, as you lose weight. Excessive hunger, cravings, or an inability to be satisfied after a meal all indicate a leptin problem. Many health problems are associated with leptin, and leptin magnifies problems that may already exist.

Leptin is not just about obesity. Anorexia and other eating disorders have links to leptin. Leptin is a critical hormone necessary for reproduction, development, puberty, and fertility. It's important for bone health and is important for people with osteoporosis or osteopenia. Leptin is important for cardiovascular health and reduces your risk of heart attacks, strokes, peripheral vascular disease, and other ailments. Leptin is important for neurological health, and its absence is linked to dementia and other cognitive impairments. Leptin is tied to the immune system and has influences on your risk for cancer.

Good Sleep Is Vital to Leptin

Have you ever felt ravenous the day after a bad night's sleep? Most people tend to overeat and gain weight during times when they do not get enough sleep. Healthy sleep is vital for leptin balance. It has been known for many years that chronic insomniacs are hungry all the time and tend to gain weight. Study after study has shown that people who sleep less weigh more. This is due mainly to hormonal imbalances caused by sleep deprivation. Poor sleep disrupts many of your hormones, insulin, thyroid hormone, growth hormone, cortisol, and others. But the disruption of natural leptin balance is the main reason that sleep deprivation causes weight gain.

Although many hormones are affected by sleep, leptin is one of the more vulnerable. Normally, leptin has a circadian rhythm. That is, it peaks at night when you sleep and is reduced during the day. This rise of leptin during the night, and its fall during the day, are natural cycles necessary for leptin balance. When the sleep cycle is disrupted, the nighttime leptin surge is blunted. This causes lower leptin levels and will make you ravenous. Even just a few nights of poor sleep can lower your leptin levels by as much as 25 percent. The decrease in leptin sends a false signal to the brain that the body is starving and needs more food.

Poor sleep also causes insulin resistance, which in turn causes leptin resistance. It's a vicious cycle, but even worse. The body's natural response to hormone resistance is to make more of the hormone, to overcome the resistance. But when your sleep is troubled, you're put at a major disadvantage because you can't ramp up leptin production when it's most needed.

To lose weight and keep it off, you must balance your hormones. Eating right and getting enough exercise simply are not enough. It's important to get sufficient sleep, but it's equally important that the sleep you are getting is quality sleep. Everyone needs a different amount of sleep, and the amount your body needs is determined largely by genetics. Studies have shown, however, that people who sleep less than five hours per night have the most severe leptin problems.

The bottom line is that if your body does not get enough sleep, or if the sleep it is getting is of poor quality, you are putting yourself at a disadvantage. Your nightly surge of leptin will be diminished and your normal circadian rhythm will be disrupted. It's just another cause of leptin imbalance, and the end result will be that you'll feel ravenous and gain weight. This is why sleep is so critical. It's just one more piece of the puzzle.

The Biology of Fat

Not all fat is the same. Different types of fat play various roles in the regulation of hormone production, heat generation, metabolism, and body weight. Fat cells vary in two ways: location and type. Fat is the only tissue in the body that has unlimited growth potential throughout your entire life.

Fat is important for regulating body temperature and metabolism. Through complex brain-hormone interactions, the body controls its own body temperature. The production of body heat is called *thermogenesis,* which is a major indicator of metabolism. Increased thermogenesis is the result of increased metabolism. It's like running an engine; the harder it runs, the hotter it gets. Low body temperature means lowered metabolism.

Fat comes in two colors, brown and white. *White adipose tissue* (WAT) is the tissue that produces hormones like leptin, adiponectin, and resistin. Body heat production occurs in brown fat tissue (also known as *brown adipose tissue*, or BAT). BAT is controlled by the brain, nerves, and stress hormones such as epinephrine and norepinephrine. A special receptor for these hormones is found only in BAT. It is called a β-3 receptor. The hormones epinephrine and norepinephrine work by stimulating b-receptors. Stimulation of the β-3 receptor increases metabolism by increasing heat production and fat breakdown. Just as healthy BAT can be part of the cycle to help lose weight, dysfunctional BAT can get in the way. If you are extremely overweight, your brown fat tissue cannot produce heat properly, so your metabolism is slow and it becomes even harder to lose weight.

Thermogenins are proteins made by brown fat tissue and are responsible for body heat production. Thermogenins are regulated by blood proteins, known as uncoupling proteins. The more uncoupling proteins you have, the higher your metabolism.

Visceral Fat

The scientific community has widely accepted the fact that body fat distribution plays a major role in the development of leptin resistance, insulin resistance, and the Metabolic Syndrome. Excess weight in the belly is the hallmark of hormone resistance. It's called central obesity, or *visceral adiposity* (*viscera* = internal organs, *adipo* = fat) because the fat lies in the midsection, surrounding the organs. Men with a waistline of more than 40 inches and women with a waistline of more than 35 inches are classified as having central obesity. But experts agree that leptin resistance and insulin resistance occur in people with even slimmer waistlines.

Visceral adipocytes—the fat cells surrounding internal organs—are responsible for hormone resistance. They are what I call *metabolically evil*. Fat in the midsection is highly active tissue that is regulated by many other hormones. Hormonal imbalance has dramatic effects on the fat cells in your belly. Increased cortisol or decreased growth hormone increases visceral adiposity; and also lowers testosterone in men and estrogen in women. Even subtle

TOXIC FAT

The term visceral adipocytes is a misnomer. Viscera refers to the belly and internal organs, although these cells are found throughout the body. The traditional view has been that toxic fat cells, or visceral adipocytes, were found only in the belly. We now know that they are also found inside muscles, including those of the heart, as well as inside organs. These fat cells are the ones that produce harmful hormones like TNF-α and IL-6, which result in leptin resistance and insulin resistance. Toxic fat buildup in organs can also lead to malfunction of the organ.

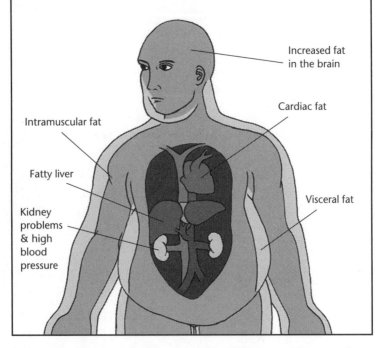

hormonal changes will start a cascade of leptin resistance and insulin resistance that promotes accumulation of fat in the belly. As visceral fat accumulates, it induces hormonal changes to grow even more visceral fat—talk about hormonal imbalance! Visceral fat slows metabolism and stimulates leptin and insulin resistance. It increases cortisol levels and lowers growth hormone levels. Visceral fat increases the risk of diabetes, high blood pressure, high triglycerides, low good cholesterol, gout, sleep apnea, fatty liver disease, and cardiovascular disease.

Visceral fat cells are in more places that we once realized. The original notion that scientists had was that these fat cells were limited to an area in the abdomen known as the omentum. It turns out, however, that visceral fat cells are located throughout the body. They are the cells that cover the heart, called pericardial fat pads. And they are found in little patches, attached to all the organs. Visceral fat cells even penetrate the organs. The liver, for example, stores a tremendous amount of fat. People with leptin resistance develop fatty liver disease as a consequence of increased visceral fat. Even people who are lean and do not have a big belly can have increased visceral fat cells from these other sources of fat. The fat that penetrates your muscles is metabolically similar to visceral fat. This fat, located far from the belly, is just as metabolically evil. It causes flabby muscles and makes people feel weak and have muscle cramps. And fat in the muscles causes the same host of metabolic derangements as does visceral fat.

So you don't have to be obese, or even have increased fat in the belly, to have too much visceral fat. Dr. Neil Rudderman has described this phenomenon as MONW—Metabolically Obese Normal Weight. This condition is associated with increased risk of cardiovascular disease and the host of ailments seen with the Metabolic Syndrome. Your body weight is only part of your challenge in achieving hormonal balance. You have to have lean, healthy muscles that are free of toxic fat cells.

We are just now beginning to understand the complex biology of visceral fat cells. We know that these cells produce more toxic hormones, known as inflammatory cytokines or adipokines such as TNF-α and IL-6. They also make more of the blood-clotting factor PAI-1, which is a mediator of cardiovascular disease. Scientists have identified receptors for cortisol and testosterone on visceral fat cells, indicating their responsiveness to these important hormones.

Peripheral Fat

The fat in your legs, in your buttocks, and under your skin is dramatically different than visceral fat and is considered "healthy" fat.

It doesn't induce the cascade of metabolic derangements seen with visceral fat. Peripheral fat makes most of your leptin and adiponectin.

The vast differences between visceral fat and peripheral fat have led some scientists to suggest that they are actually two separate endocrine organs. It makes sense, considering that visceral fat produces harmful inflammatory adipokines while peripheral fat makes healthy fat hormones like leptin and adiponectin. Two different types of fat are serving the role of two different glands. Under normal circumstances, the two types of fat work together to balance malnutrition and obesity and to keep your weight normal. We all have both visceral fat *and* peripheral fat. When your hormones are balanced, the peripheral fat dominates and visceral fat is kept to a minimum.

Adipokines—Inflammation Hormones

Macrophages are specialized cells that are designed to kill invaders. They produce toxic chemicals, known as cytokines, which fight infections and cancer. Macrophages are actually a type of white blood cell, but they are found in virtually every organ. When they take up residence in an organ, they begin to alter its function. Macrophages migrate toward fat cells, and in particular they love to intermix with visceral fat cells. Macrophages become integrated with visceral fat tissue, and their activity is considered part of the glandular activity of fat. So it's not just the traditional fat cells, or adipocytes, that make hormones. These fat macrophages are also major players in the endocrinology of fat. When fat tissue produces inflammatory cytokines, they are called adipokines. The two most important of these are TNF-α and IL-6.

Tumor Necrosis Factor-Alpha

TNF-α, tumor necrosis factor, is a cytokine hormone that was first described because of its ability to cause necrosis, or breakdown of tumors. It was later shown to be identical to *cachexin*, a substance secreted by white blood cells that was considered responsible for the loss of appetite and weight loss seen in patients with advanced cancer. Although first studied in cancer patients, TNF-α is now thought to play a major role in the development of leptin resistance, insulin resistance, obesity, and an increased risk of cardiovascular disease.

In some ways, TNF-α is beneficial. It fights infections and cancer cells. It decreases appetite and increases the production of leptin. The problem is that the detrimental effects of TNF-α outweigh its benefits. TNF-α is a toxic hormone. It causes inflammation, which is a major cause of hormone resistance. When you have excess fat in the belly, excess TNF-α induces leptin resistance and insulin resistance. TNF-α also increases cortisol levels, another cause of excess fat in the belly. So even though TNF-α decreases appetite and boosts leptin production, these effects can be overwhelmed by its more potent effect of causing resistance to both leptin and insulin. The end result: increased appetite and slower metabolism.

Interleukin-6

IL-6, or interleukin-6, is a cytokine hormone that's closely associated with obesity, leptin resistance, and insulin resistance. Interleukins are chemical messengers made by white blood cells, or *leukocytes* (*inter* = communication, *leuko* = white blood cell). At least 18 types of interleukins are known. They have a variety of roles in the body, involving inflammation and the immune system. IL-6 is the interleukin made by a specialized type of white blood cell known as macrophages, discussed earlier. Macrophages love to infiltrate fat. These white blood cells integrate with the fat cells and become part of the fat as a functioning unit. When scientists study fat hormones, they find it difficult to tell whether a particular hormone is coming from fat cells themselves or from the macrophages infiltrated in between the fat. The macrophages are considered part of the fat as it functions as a glandular organ. Macrophages are part of the larger picture, yet an important part. Researchers have targeted macrophages as possibly being a key to unlock the secrets of adipokines and inflammation and to learn how they cause obesity and cardiovascular disease.

While all fat makes IL-6, visceral fat, primarily because of its abundance of macrophages, makes three to four times as much IL-6 compared to peripheral fat. The higher your IL-6 levels, the greater your chance of having resistance to leptin and insulin. Increased IL-6 levels have been correlated with an increased risk for diabetes and cardiovascular disease. When you lose weight, one of the first things to happen is that your IL-6 levels go down.

Leptin Is a Cytokine Hormone

Amazingly, the chemical structure of leptin is very similar to that of inflammatory cytokines like TNF-α and IL-6. And the leptin receptor's structure is almost identical to that of cytokine receptors. They are all part of one big cytokine "superfamily." At first, this was a surprise to scientists, because leptin acts so differently than cytokines. But this is not unusual with hormones. Hormones that are quite similar in structure can have dramatically opposite actions. This is because they may be similar enough to be attracted to the same receptor, but different enough that one turns on the receptor while the other turns it off. The fact is that the cytokine hormones—TNF-α, IL-6, and leptin—all decrease appetite. The difference is that TNF-α and IL-6 also cause inflammation and leptin resistance, cancelling out the effect on appetite.

The Key to Leptin Action— NF Kappa β and Jak-Stat Pathways

All hormones work by inducing a series of events inside a cell. The science that studies these microcellular changes is truly cutting edge. This is where the real science is happening today. Every time I attend a scientific meeting, I hear about more and more attention being paid to the intricate pathways that occur inside cells.

Hormones bind with their receptor and induce two major pathways in the cells. One is called NF kappa β, and the other Jak-Stat. These molecules help hormones work by acting as a mediator between the hormone receptor and the DNA. These two pathways are thought to be the underlying mechanism for leptin problems. The Jak-Stat pathway is responsible for leptin action. The NF kappa β pathway is responsible for leptin resistance and other types of hormone resistance. Once researchers better understand these pathways, new treatments for leptin resistance and obesity are likely to emerge.

NF kappa β, or *nuclear factor-kappa beta,* is the basis of both inflammation and aging. Research is focused on methods of suppressing this lethal agent as a way of protecting against many age-related diseases. NF kappa β has been linked to obesity and degenerative conditions like arthritis, cancer, asthma, Alzheimer's, osteoporosis, cardiovascular disease, and diabetes. In the most basic terms, NF kappa β is a protein that turns on inflammation like you flip a light switch. Some researchers believe that inflammation is at the core of 98 percent of human disease, so this makes NF kappa β a highly important molecule. Antioxidants inhibit it, which is why diets high in fruits and vegetables are so good at preventing inflammation. Vitamins E and C and omega-3 fatty acids have been shown to inhibit production of NF kappa β. Other agents that may have a beneficial effect include curcumin (the primary ingredient in curry seasoning), soy products, hot peppers, basil, rosemary, ginger, and pomegranates.

The Janus kinase (JAK) and signal transducers and activator of transcription (STAT) proteins, called Jak-Stat for short, are mediators important to the action of cytokine hormones. Leptin is a cytokine hormone that works through this pathway, but so do TNF-α and IL-6. Various cytokine hormones have actions through the same Jak-Stat pathway.

The New Fat Cell Hormones

Leptin's discovery led to the understanding that fat cells are more than merely a passive reservoir for energy storage. It opened the eyes of obesity researchers, revealing that the fat cells are a highly active hormone-producing tissue. Once scientists realized that fat cells made leptin, they set out to discover other fat cell hormones. White adipose tissue is now recognized to be a multifunctional organ; in addition to its central role of storing fat, it has a major endocrine function of secreting several hormones. It was previously known that fat cells made cytokine hormones like TNF-α and IL-6. These fat cell hormones have been given the name *adipocytokines* or *adipokines*. But now even *more* fat cell hormones have been discovered. Adiponectin, resistin, visfatin, apelin, and plasminogen activator inhibitor-1 are only a few of the important new fat cell hormones that have potent effects on appetite, metabolism, body weight, and risk for cardiovascular disease. Fat tissue is also a major site where testosterone, estrogen, and cortisol are metabolized. The importance of these endocrine functions of fat is emphasized by pondering the adverse metabolic consequences of excess visceral fat. To have hormonal balance, all your fat cell hormones must be balanced.

FAT CELL HORMONES	
Beneficial Hormones	**Detrimental Hormones**
Leptin	TNF-α
Adiponectin	IL-6
Visfatin	Resistin
Apelin	RELM-α
	Pref-1
	MCP-1
	RBP4
	ASP

Adiponectin

One beneficial fat cell hormone, adiponectin, has anti-inflammatory properties as well as the ability to lower blood sugar and reverse leptin resistance and insulin resistance. Adiponectin reduces appetite and raises metabolism. Adiponectin exerts a protective effect on blood vessels, lowering the risk of cardiovascular disease. Low levels of it are associated with leptin resistance, insulin resistance, metabolic syndrome, obesity, heart attacks, and strokes. Although adiponectin was discovered after leptin, much of today's research is focused on it as a key to curing obesity. Since its discovery, thousands of scientific articles have been published on adiponectin.

Adiponectin is made primarily by your healthy, peripheral fat. Unhealthy, visceral fat cells aren't able to make much adiponectin, because they are preoccupied with making the toxic hormones TNF-α and IL-6. Receptors for adiponectin are located mostly in muscle tissue, vascular tissue, and the liver. Adiponectin exerts its beneficial effects by improving the way these organs function. In the liver, adiponectin reduces the production of sugar and free fatty acids. In blood vessels, adiponectin protects from damage and injury. In muscles, it enhances their ability to take in glucose, decreasing insulin resistance and making a stronger, metabolically healthy muscle.

Adiponectin production is increased by stimulation of the PPAR-gamma receptor, the site of action of the diabetes medications rosiglitazone (Avandia) and pioglitazone (Actos). I'll talk more about these medications in Chapter 15.

Adiponectin decreases leptin resistance and insulin resistance, in part because of its anti-inflammatory properties. Research shows that adiponectin is a unique fat cell hormone with a variety of effects that promote health. Early tests have shown that when adiponectin is given to animals, they have lower blood sugar, lower triglycerides, and less insulin resistance.

Even though adiponectin is made by fat cells, the heavier you are, the less adiponectin you make. It's a paradox that initially surprised researchers. It's just the opposite of leptin, which increases as you get heavier. A defect in the gene for adiponectin is thought to be one of the causes of Metabolic Syndrome. A genetically bred mouse that produces excessive amounts of adiponectin is less susceptible to cardiovascular disease, diabetes, and other ailments of Western society.

When you boost your leptin, you get an added benefit of boosting adiponectin as well. The Leptin Boost Diet will help your peripheral fat cells be strong and efficient to produce ample amounts of adiponectin, keeping your body lean and healthy.

Visfatin

In 2005, Japanese researchers identified a fat cell hormone called visfatin. Its discovery has increased the complexity of fat cell biology, because it happens to be a beneficial fat cell hormone. The unique thing about it is that it is produced by visceral fat cells—the same cells that make toxic cytokine hormones like TNF-α and IL-6. Interestingly, visfatin is also a cytokine hormone. It just goes to show how complicated things can be. Throughout this book, I've been telling you about how visceral fat cells produce toxic hormones, but visfatin is an exception to that rule.

Visfatin is important for the regulation of appetite, metabolism, and body weight. It is also linked to the development of insulin resistance, diabetes, and the Metabolic Syndrome. The more visceral fat you have, the more visfatin you make. It is known as an "insulin mimetic" because it acts in a similar way to insulin. It stimulates the insulin receptor, helping lower blood sugar and reducing insulin resistance. When blood sugar levels are high, visfatin is released. People with diabetes have lower visfatin levels, giving credence to the belief that a deficiency of this hormone contributes to the development of diabetes. The brain also contains visfatin receptors, and in the same location as leptin receptors. It is thought that visfatin works in a similar way to leptin in the brain, instead signaling the body about the amount of fat your body is storing.

Apelin

Another adipokine hormone made by fat cells is called apelin. As with leptin, apelin levels go up as you gain weight. Insulin resistance and high insulin levels will stimulate fat cells to make more apelin. Apelin is thought to be a beneficial fat cell hormone. In the cardiovascular system, apelin relaxes blood vessels and reduces blood pressure. In addition, apelin has been demonstrated to make the heart beat stronger, even when the heart muscle has been injured.

Resistin

Named because of its ability to cause insulin resistance, resistin is another cytokine hormone made by fat cells. The more visceral fat you have, the more resistin you make. Resistin has major effects on the blood vessels and is thought to contribute to the formation of atherosclerosis and cardiovascular disease.

Resistin-Like Molecule Alpha

One hormone made by adipose tissue, resistin-like molecule alpha (RELM-α), is thought to have actions similar to those of resistin. A similar hormone, RELM-β, is made by the gastrointestinal tract, particularly the colon.

Preadipocyte Factor-1

The fat cell hormone called preadipocyte factor-1 (Pref-1) is involved in the formation of fat cells, a process known as adipogenesis. It's primarily made by immature fat cells, known as *preadipocytes*. High levels of Pref-1 cause insulin resistance.

Plasminogen Activator Inhibitor-1

A substance that stops the breakdown of blood clots, PAI-1, or plasminogen activator inhibitor-1, is not officially a hormone, but rather a protein made by fat cells. By slowing the resolution of a clot, PAI-1 makes your body more susceptible to cardiovascular disease. It's considered a major risk for heart attacks and strokes and is now tested for, just like cholesterol and triglycerides. Increased circulating levels of PAI-1 are common in the Metabolic Syndrome and contribute to an associated risk of elevated cardiovascular problems. The lining of the blood vessels, known as the endothelium, is also a major producer of PAI-1. If you have increased fat in the belly, your PAI-1 levels will go up, and so will your risk of cardiovascular disease. PAI-1 is related to the development of obesity. Research on an inhibitor of PAI-1 given to mice fed a high-fat diet resulted in a reduced weight gain and an improved metabolism.

Monocyte Chemoattractant Protein–1

The hormone called MCP-1, or monocyte chemoattractant protein–1, is made by fat cells, white blood cells, and blood vessel cells. This hormone attracts specialized white blood cells known as monocytes and macrophages. These cells are mediators of atherosclerosis and cardiovascular disease. MCP-1 attracts macrophages to infiltrate fat tissue. Macrophages that have infiltrated fat are the major producers of the toxic cytokines TNF-α and IL-6.

The heavier you are, the higher your MCP-1 levels. MCP-1 is also increased by leptin resistance. MCP-1 links obesity and insulin resistance by causing inflammation. MCP-1 is also thought to be involved in the development of fatty liver disease, a complication of obesity and leptin resistance.

Retinol-Binding Protein 4

Retinol-Binding Protein 4 (RBP4) is a protein, produced by fat cells, that is closely associated with obesity, insulin resistance, prediabetes, and type 2 diabetes. Elevated RPB4 levels are linked to a high risk of cardiovascular disease and Metabolic Syndrome. Researchers have suggested that measuring RPB4 levels could be a good test to assess someone's risk for diabetes or cardiovascular disease. Research has also been conducted on ways to decrease RPB4 as a means of reducing insulin resistance and preventing these diseases.

Acylation-Stimulating Protein

The hormone called acylation-stimulating protein (ASP) is made by fat cells and in turn stimulates the growth and production of new fat cells. Not much is known about this hormone, but it is believed to act as a bridge for fat cells to communicate with each other.

3

BRAIN HORMONES

The Brain Is a Gland

The nervous system is an important part of the endocrine system, both producing hormones and responding to other hormones. The hunger center in the brain, located in the hypothalamus, is the main site of action for leptin, adiponectin, and other hunger hormones. This part of the brain not only responds to hormones but actually makes dozens, if not hundreds, of its own hunger hormones, all of which have varying effects on your appetite. Brain hormones may be called neurotransmitters, proteins, neuropeptides, molecules, or cytokines. But regardless of the name, they are all potent hormones that are critical components of your appetite control system. Fat cells have the biological inventory needed for storing and releasing energy, but adipose tissue also contains hormonal systems that permit communication with the central nervous system. Through these interactions, fat tissue is integrally involved in coordinating appetite, metabolism, energy levels, and immune function.

The hypothalamus, the main appetite center in the brain, is the same region of the brain that controls the pituitary gland. Brain cells, known as neurons, in the hypothalamus have receptors for fat cell hormones and are able to respond at a moment's notice. Leptin, for example, has receptors on two types of brain cells that, in turn, produce the brain hormones that control hunger and appetite. It's all a big chain of hormonal events. Hormones made by your fat tell your brain to make more hormones. Then these hormones tell the rest of the body to make even *more* hormones. Along the way, these hormones have a variety of effects on your appetite, level of satisfaction with a meal, cravings, metabolism, and body weight. It can get pretty complicated.

Neurons in the appetite control center produce hormonal substances like POMC, neuropeptide Y, endocannabinoids, and many others that are the underlying regulators of appetite and body weight. Hormones like leptin influence your appetite through these neuropeptide mediators. The brain functions as the body's biological control center, constantly sensing your body's nutritional status. It works like the conductor of this vast symphony of hunger hormones, responding to hormones and in turn making its own hormones. The brain is intimately involved in all of this. You can't talk about leptin (or about any other hunger hormones, for that matter) without talking about the brain.

The site of action for leptin, adiponectin, and other fat cell hormones is largely confined to the hypothalamus—the appetite control center. This is where fat cell hormones direct the production of more hormones. Leptin, for example, has its receptors on neurons that make POMC and neuropeptide Y (NPY). These brain hormones have long-term effects on food intake and body weight. Neuropeptide Y is a hormone that increases food intake and is decreased by leptin. POMC is a hormone that decreases food intake and is increased by leptin.

The blood-brain barrier is a membrane that controls the passage of substances that cross from the bloodstream into the brain. The blood-brain barrier lies between blood vessels and critical parts of the brain. It is nature's way of acting as a gatekeeper for substances entering the brain. Many of the problems with fat cell hormones involve the blood-brain barrier. Leptin, for example, can have difficulties penetrating the barrier. When this occurs, leptin can't enter the brain and can't pass its signals on to NPY and POMC. It is thought that many problems in the research on giving leptin injections for weight loss occurred because synthetic leptin could not cross the blood-brain barrier. There is ongoing research on producing a form of synthetic leptin that will easily cross that barrier.

Appetite is also affected by other hormones, including metabolic hormones and those produced by the digestive tract, such as

LEPTIN'S EFFECT ON BRAIN HORMONES

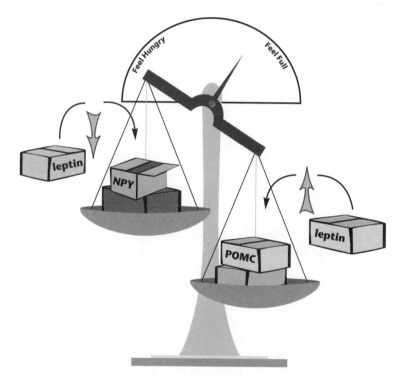

Leptin works via two brain hormones—POMC and NPY. These hormones ultimately regulate appetite and body weight. Most of your leptin receptors are found on neurons that produce these important brain hormones. NPY is a potent stimulator of appetite, while POMC has the opposite effect. Leptin works to decrease NPY and increase POMC production. When your hormones are balanced, this appetite control system helps to keep your body weight in the normal range. Hormonal imbalance, including leptin resistance, will lead to increased NPY levels, decreased POMC, and increased appetite. Boosting leptin decreases NPY and increases POMC, lessening appetite and augmenting metabolism.

cholecystokinin, glucagon-like peptide-1, and ghrelin. I'll talk more about these hormones in the following chapters.

Proopiomelanocortin

POMC, proopiomelanocortin, is critical to the action of leptin. Neurons that produce POMC are covered with receptors for leptin. When leptin is acting in the brain, POMC is one of the more important mediators. POMC is a hormone that's known as a *prohormone* because the body breaks it apart into smaller parts, many of which have diverse hormonal activities. It's an important hormone in the obesity saga and is greatly influenced both by leptin and by other hormones.

POMC AND ITS COMPONENTS

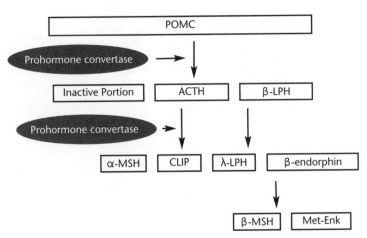

POMC is a large hormone produced by the hypothalamus and pituitary gland. This inactive hormone is broken apart by special enzymes, including prohormone convertase, into smaller, active hormones, including ACTH and α-MSH, both of which are important hormones related to leptin and overall body weight.

In a research setting, mice that have a defective gene for POMC weigh twice as much as normal mice. POMC-deficient mice eat all the time and yet, on the surface, appear similar to the obese, leptin-deficient mouse.

POMC is made by both the pituitary gland and the hypothalamus. In the pituitary gland, POMC is turned into the cortisol-regulating hormone called ACTH. ACTH can be processed further to alpha melanocyte-stimulating hormone, or α-MSH, a potent hormone that shuts down appetite. It's known as an *anorectic neuropeptide*, because it causes *anorexia*, or loss of appetite. If you don't have enough α-MSH, you'll be hungry all the time.

α-MSH deficiency, caused by problems processing POMC, has been identified in humans. It's caused by a defective substance known as *prohormone convertase*. If you don't have prohormone convertase, you can't break apart POMC and you can't make the α-MSH you need to keep your appetite under control. People with this genetic defect become very obese at an early age and have red hair. The α-MSH deficiency causes the red hair because the hormone has a second function of stimulating pigment-producing cells known as melanocytes (hence its original name—melanocyte stimulating factor). If your prohormone convertase doesn't work, you'll also have adrenal insufficiency, known as Addison's disease, due to a lack of ACTH. For more information on ACTH and the adrenal gland, please see Chapter 6.

The receptor for α-MSH is known as the *MCR-4 receptor*. Research indicates that as many as 4 percent of people who have severe obesity may have a mutation of this receptor. Up to 6 percent of severely obese children have a mutated MCR-4 receptor. Close to 30 percent of all Americans are candidates for having MCR-4 mutations. It is the most common *single gene mutation* linked to obesity. The MCR-4 receptor has become a very important target in current obesity research. It all goes back to leptin. Leptin stimulates POMC, which breaks apart to α-MSH, which stimulates the MCR-4 receptor.

The first report of a naturally obese mouse was in 1902, as detailed earlier. French geneticist L. Cuenot described an obese yellow mouse now known as the *agouti* mouse, which had a bright yellow coat color and obesity proportional to the yellow coat's intensity.

The brighter the yellow coat, the more obese the mouse. It's now known that this mouse has too much of a substance known as agouti. Agouti is a protein that blocks binding of α-MSH to the melanocortin-4 receptor. So agouti is a bad thing. To much of it means that MCR-4 won't work. If MCR-4 doesn't work, then leptin can't function properly.

MSH AND THE MCR4 RECEPTOR

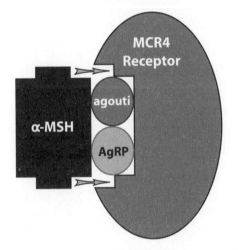

Leptin works by stimulating α-MSH production. α-MSH works via the MCR4 receptor. Substances known as agouti and agouti-related protein (AgRP) block the MCR-4 receptor, rendering α-MSH ineffective. If leptin does not work properly, there will be too little α-MSH. As many as 3 to 4 percent of severely obese humans have a defective MCR4 receptor. Problems with too little α-MSH, too much agouti or agouti-related protein, or a defective MCR4 receptor not only will cause obesity, but will cause an individual to have red hair.

Researchers found that destruction of the outer regions of the hypothalamus in these mice caused loss of appetite, due to the destruction of nerve cells containing appetite-stimulating neurotransmitters. *Agouti-related protein (AgRP)* is a substance that works like agouti. Too much agouti-related protein causes hunger and weight gain. AgRP is an important and very active area in obesity research.

LEPTIN AND BEYOND: WHERE THINGS CAN GO WRONG

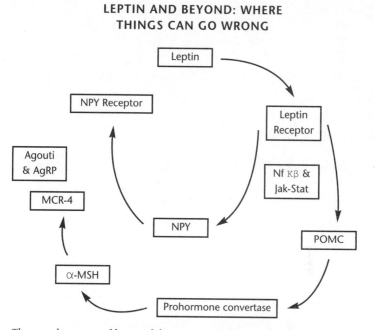

There can be many problems with leptin. Leptin deficiency is very rare, but a problem with the way leptin works and the cascade of other hormones it influences is vast. The discovery of leptin has unlocked the secrets to a multitude of hunger hormones that have become the targets of cutting-edge obesity research today.

Neuropeptide Y

NPY, or neuropeptide Y, is the most potent stimulator of appetite known to humans. NPY is a brain hormone that is directly influenced by leptin. Normally, leptin keeps NPY levels low. Neuropeptide Y has many different actions on the hypothalamus as well as other areas of the brain and body. It increases appetite and stimulates the accumulation of body fat.

When leptin drops, or if you develop leptin resistance, NPY levels go up. Increased NPY increases production of ACTH, which then stimulates the adrenal gland to make too much cortisol. Excess cortisol further increases appetite and causes leptin resistance. So any imbalance of NPY leads to disruptions of your entire appetite control system.

Serotonin

One brain chemical that makes the body feel good is serotonin. It has effects on your hunger, sleep, anxiety level, and mood. If your serotonin level is low, you will feel hungry, anxious, and depressed. Serotonin is also the hormone responsible for carbohydrate cravings. It's the reason why you reach for the bag of pretzels or a candy bar in the late afternoon.

Serotonin has led to a greater understanding of depression and a class of medications known as selective serotonin reuptake inhibitors (SSRIs)—antidepressant drugs like Lexapro, Celexa, Prozac, Zoloft, Paxil, and Remeron. Serotonin is a brain chemical that is critical in the regulation of hunger, appetite, and carbohydrate cravings.

Leptin resistance can cause your brain to not produce enough serotonin.

SSRIs also have a double effect on your weight. They can cause either weight loss or weight gain. In my experience, I have seen that Prozac and Zoloft usually cause weight loss in the first six months and then cause weight gain. Paxil and Remeron are more likely to cause weight gain from the start. SSRIs have similarities to prescription diet pills like Meridia and phentermine.

Serotonin, norepinephrine, and dopamine are all interrelated when it comes to weight. Antidepressant medications like venlafaxine (Effexor) and duloxetine (Cymbalta) work by increasing levels of these three brain hormones. This combination approach is better for weight loss. Patients who take these medications report modest weight loss. Meridia is a cousin of these medications. This weight-loss medication reports an average loss of 25 pounds in six months' time. If the medication is discontinued, however, the weight is regained.

St. John's Wort is a nutritional supplement that increases serotonin levels. It has been advertised as a natural remedy for depression, anxiety, and obesity. Studies on St. John's Wort have not been positive. It appears that St. John's Wort is not very effective for weight loss and can have potentially dangerous side effects.

Serotonin receptor 2c (known in scientific terms as 5-HT 2c) is a specialized receptor responsible for the appetite and carbohydrate-craving effects of serotonin. These receptors are found in the hypothalamus—now familiar as our appetite control center. When this receptor is stimulated, hunger is reduced. The weight-loss medication Meridia works via the 5-HT 2c receptor. If you can't properly stimulate this receptor, you are hungry all the time and have carbohydrate cravings. Antidepressant medications can make you gain weight or lose weight. Their effect is through this receptor as well.

When the 5-HT 2c receptor doesn't work properly, it sets in motion a flood of hormonal imbalance that perpetuates weight gain. Problems with the 5-HT 2c receptor cause leptin resistance. It's another vicious cycle.

Dopamine

The role of dopamine in the hormonal control of obesity remains controversial. Scientists know that destruction of the outer regions of the hypothalamus in mice causes loss of appetite, due to the destruction of nerve cells containing the appetite-stimulating brain hormones like dopamine. By contrast, medications that increase dopamine increase appetite. The antidepressant medication *bupropion* (Wellbutrin) affects both the norepinephrine and the dopamine systems and causes weight loss.

Gamma-Aminobutyric Acid

GABA, or gamma-aminobutyric acid, is a brain hormone linked to appetite and obesity. Leptin resistance increases GABA levels. GABA is increased by prescription antianxiety medications that have weight gain as a side effect. Benzodiazepine medications like Xanax, Valium, and Librium relieve anxiety and make you sleepy by stimulating the GABA receptor. The medications Topamax and Zonegran are traditionally used to treat seizures and migraine headaches and work by decreasing GABA. These medications also decrease appetite and stop overeating. These medications are very useful in reducing binge eating and eating at night. Although these medications are not yet approved for the treatment of weight loss, I have treated many patients with them and have seen some amazing results. Several of my patients have lost over one hundred pounds from taking Topamax. I'll discuss these medications in more detail in Chapter 15.

Endocannabinoids

The brain produces its own set of compounds, known as endo-cannabinoids, that are similar to marijuana, The active component of marijuana, tetrahydrocannabinol, was identified in the 1960s. This compound causes increased appetite in people who smoke marijuana. It's known as the "munchies." Endocannabinoids do the same thing—they increase appetite.

The first endocannabinoid was named *anandamide*, from the Sanskrit word ananda for "bliss." Receptors for endocannabinoids are found in the appetite control center of the brain. Marinol is a marijuana-like medication used to increase appetite and relieve nausea. Rimonabant (Acomplia) is a medication that works by blocking the actions of endocannabinoids. It causes weight loss by decreasing appetite and cravings.

Cocaine- and Amphetamine-Related Transcript

Both cocaine and amphetamines are known to be potent, appetite-suppressant drugs. People who use these stimulants lose weight. This knowledge has led to the discovery of *cocaine and amphetamine-related transcript,* or CART, a brain hormone involved in appetite, reward, and reinforcement. Not much is known about CART, but it's thought to hold promise as a potential area to target for future obesity research.

Galanin

The brain hormone galanin stimulates appetite and raises blood sugar levels. It also increases levels of growth hormone. Additionally, galanin is involved in reward and pleasure centers in the brain and has been linked to some of the addictive properties of junk food and fast food, both of which can act like heroin or cocaine.

4

GUT HORMONES

Short-Term Appetite Control

Hormonal signaling is critical for all aspects of life. Your stomach and intestines are no exception. The gastrointestinal tract makes hormones that communicate with the brain to tell it how full you are. This brain-gut connection is important for telling the body to stop eating. Gut hormones tell the brain about your moment-to-moment nutritional status, and not as much about how overweight or underweight you are. When your stomach is full, gut hormones are affected. This is a very different situation than with leptin and other fat cell hormones, which are more interested in the body's fat stores and overall nutritional status than the short-term swings of meals going through the digestive tract.

Every time you eat, a chemical reaction takes place between your hormones and the food. Hormones control your gut, and, in turn, your gut produces hormones. These hormones control your moment-to-moment appetite and cravings. Gut hormones respond to two main things—how much food you eat, and the content of the food. When the stomach and intestines swell with food, gut hormones are released. Regardless of the type of food, if there is a lot of it, the stretching of the stomach induces cells to make hormones (or, in the case of ghrelin, to stop making hormones). The stretch-

GUT HORMONES

Stomach hormones' response to food in your stomach

Full Stomach   Empty Stomach

Gut hormones respond to short-term changes inside your stomach and intestines. Stomach distention as well as the content of particular foods (protein and fat, for example) influence gut hormones, which in turn have powerful effects on our hunger and cravings. When food enters the gut, levels of ghrelin (a potent, appetite-stimulating hormone) decrease and levels of cholecystokinin, glucagon-like peptide-1, and peptide YY (appetite-reducing hormones) go up.

ing effect is short lived, and the effect of gut hormones on your appetite can be equally short-lived.

To take advantage of gut hormones, you have to be able to keep them going for as long as possible. Good ways to do this are to eat frequently throughout the day and to eat large amounts of low-calorie foods. This is why foods that are high in volume but low in calories are so great for weight loss. Foods like fruits, vegetables, and other high-fiber foods swell in the stomach, thereby stimulating gut hormone production and shutting down appetite.

The composition of the food in your meal will also affect your gut hormones. The hormone most closely linked to food is insulin. But insulin mostly responds to the amount and type of carbohydrates in your meal. Insulin isn't the only hormone affected by food, nor is it necessarily the most important. Ghrelin, GLP-1, CCK, and PYY will respond to the protein and fat in your diet. Protein and fat are excellent for stimulating gut hormones (and suppressing ghrelin) for longer periods. This is why I recommend that you eat protein in the morning. When you do so, your gut hormones go into overdrive, keeping hunger at a minimum all day long.

Ghrelin

Ghrelin is a hormone released from cells in the lining of the stomach and in the intestinal tract. This hormone is a potent stimulator of appetite. If your ghrelin levels are high, you never feel full. Ghrelin works by increasing levels of NPY, the same hunger hormone that leptin works to keep down. When ghrelin rises, appetite increases. Ghrelin levels rapidly decline after meals, signaling the brain that your stomach is full.

Ghrelin's actions are the opposite of leptin's. Ghrelin stimulates appetite through production of the NPY, while leptin reduces appetite, in part, through decreasing NPY.

A genetic condition called Prader-Willi Syndrome is characterized by mental retardation and extreme hunger. Children become very obese and eat virtually everything in sight. The parents usually have to lock up all the food in the house. It turns out that children with Prader-Willi Syndrome have very high ghrelin levels.

Gastric bypass surgery is associated with a profound reduction in ghrelin levels. This decrease may account for some of the reduced hunger reported by patients who have had weight-loss surgery.

The best way to keep ghrelin levels low is to eat large volumes of low-calorie foods frequently during the day. This stretches stomach fibers, which send signals to shut down ghrelin-producing cells. It makes sense; your stomach is simply telling your brain that it is full. The brain responds by shutting down appetite. There can be lag time, however. If you eat very quickly, you will still feel hungry even though your belly is full. If you start feeling that your belly is full, stop eating, even if you still feel hungry. In a few minutes, your brain will catch up to your belly. Once ghrelin production shuts down, your appetite will subside.

Incretins

The newly discovered hormones called incretins are made by the gut and released in response to food, to enhance insulin production and decrease glucagon release. Incretin hormones help the body process food by stimulating the pancreas to produce insulin. The *incretin effect* is a phenomenon seen when researchers compare the body's hormonal response to sugar that is consumed by mouth with sugar given by injection straight into the bloodstream. When you eat a meal, incretin hormones stimulate insulin production much more than if the same nutrients were given by vein, bypassing the gut. Patients with type 2 diabetes have an impaired incretin effect.

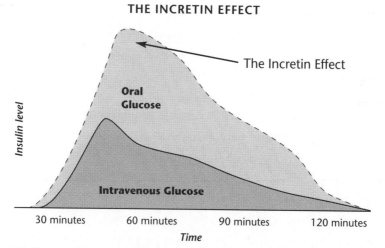

THE INCRETIN EFFECT

The "Incretin Effect" is a phenomenon seen when oral glucose administration is compared to that of intravenous glucose. The latter stimulates insulin production by β-cells in the pancreas. The same amount of glucose taken by mouth has a double effect on insulin production. When glucose or other nutrients enter the gut, they stimulate the release of incretin hormones, which increase insulin production beyond what is seen when glucose is given intravenously.

There are two major incretin hormones: glucagon-like-peptide-1 (GLP-1—pronounced "glip-one") and glucose dependant insulinotropic peptide (also know as GIP). Both GLP-1 and GIP tell the pancreas to ramp up insulin production. These hormones are made by the digestive tract in response to food and are necessary for the maintenance of appetite and blood sugar levels. When incretins go low, you feel hungry and gain weight. Receptors for incretins are found in the appetite control center of the brain.

Glucagon-like-peptide-1

An incretin hormone called glucagon-like-peptide-1 (GLP-1) is made by special cells in the gut known as *L-cells*. GLP-1 regulates appetite, satiety, blood sugar levels, and the speed of your digestive tract. GLP-1 slows the digestive tract and reduces hunger and helps you to feel more full and satisfied with a meal. It also stimulates insulin production and shuts down glucagon production. When GLP-1 levels are normal, your appetite is normal; if levels drop, you feel ravenous. Leptin resistance causes GLP-1 levels to decrease dramatically. This leads to increased hunger and weight gain.

Two approaches have been developed to harness the power of GLP-1. The first is the use of the medication exenatide (Byetta), which is known as an incretin mimetic because it imitates the way GLP-1 works. Exenatide cannot be taken in pill form or the stomach will simply digest it. It must be injected. This medication has become very widely used as a treatment for diabetes because it has a side effect of weight loss. For more information on exenatide, please see Chapter 15.

The second approach is the use of another class of drugs, known as *glipins*, which work by decreasing the breakdown of natural incretins. These drugs, vildagliptin (Galvus) and sitagliptin (Januvia)—both also called dipeptidyl peptidase-4 (DPP-4) inhibitors—reduce the breakdown of incretins, increasing the levels of natural GLP-1 and GIP. DPP-4 inhibitors tap the wisdom of the body, taking advantage of what it normally does. We do not yet understand the full importance of incretin hormones. The development of exenatide and DPP-4 inhibitors opens the door for a whole new generation of diabetes and weight-loss medications.

Glucose Dependant Insulinotropic Peptide

Formerly known as gastric inhibitory peptide, glucose dependant insulinotropic peptide (GIP) is another incretin hormone that's closely related to GLP-1. GIP is made by specialized cells in the gut known as *K-cells*. It gets its name because it stimulates the body to make insulin. Like GLP-1, GIP is released by the gut in response to a meal. Unlike GLP-1, GIP doesn't have much of an effect on glucagon.

Cholecystokinin

CCK, or cholecystokinin, is one of the body's most powerful anti-hunger hormones. It's made by the intestinal tract and released after a meal, especially one high in protein or fat. When CCK is high, it tells the brain that you are full. It's one of the main ways the gut communicates with the brain. A tremendous amount of research is now under way on CCK and how it regulates appetite and weight. Some reports show that L-phenylalanine supplementation will increase CCK levels. The problem with CCK is that it's a short-term hormone. Like other gut hormones, it's released in response to food. After the food is digested, CCK levels go back down. The effect of CCK is very short-lived.

There are two ways to stimulate CCK production, and they are the same ways that you get your body to shut down ghrelin production: eating a lot of food, or eating food high in protein or fat. Filling your belly with food, whether it is healthy food or unhealthy food, causes hormone-producing cells to make more CCK. Once the food starts getting digested and the swelling subsides, CCK production goes back down. Protein and fat have a more long-lasting effect on

CCK, which explains why they help you feel full longer than carbohydrates. The Leptin Boost Diet will help you get the most out of your CCK.

Peptide YY

PYY, or peptide YY, is a hormone produced by the digestive tract that communicates with the brain. It's a very important hormone related to appetite and satiety. When your stomach and intestines become distended from a meal, they release PYY into the circulation where it communicates with the appetite control center to shut down hunger. In 2002, scientists reported that they had found a way to shut down hunger by giving injections of the PYY hormone. Other studies, however, have not shown this effect. PYY remains an active but controversial area in obesity research.

Pancreatic Hormones

The pancreas produces many hormones that influence your appetite, the most well known being insulin. Specialized cells, called the *islets of Langerhans*, produce hormones that have potent effects on blood sugar, appetite, and metabolism. Three important pancreatic hormones are glucagon, somatostatin, and amylin. Pancreatic hormones are closely related to the food you eat and have a powerful effect on your appetite.

Glucagon

Produced by special cells in the pancreas known as α-cells (alpha-cells), glucagon is also known as a counter-insulin hormone because it makes blood sugar go up. Glucagon is a digestive hormone that is released when food—especially protein—leaves the stomach and enters the gut. Glucagon slows down the digestion of food in the stomach, helping you feel full.

People with diabetes may carry a syringe of glucagon in case of low blood sugar. A shot of glucagon will immediately raise blood sugar by causing the liver to pump out glucose. In rare cases tumors produce too much glucagon. These are called glucagonomas and their symptoms are elevated blood sugars and an itchy red rash.

Glucagon is most well known because of its cousin, glucagon-like pepdide-1 (GLP-1). The diabetes medication exenatide works like GLP-1 and helps people lose weight. One of the main actions of GLP-1 is to decrease glucagon levels.

Somatostatin

Special cells in the pancreas, known as δ-cells (delta-cells), make the hormone somatostatin. One of its main functions is to block the secretion of insulin and glucagon. Somatostatin shuts down both α-cells and β-cells. It has been studied as a weight-loss medication for children who become obese from brain damage to the appetite control centers.

Amylin

Another hormone produced by the pancreas is amylin. It is made by β-cells, which are the same cells that produce insulin. Until recently, no one knew much about amylin except that it is produced and released from the pancreas just like insulin. Anytime insulin is released, amylin is also released. A synthetic variety of amylin is now available as a medication known as pramlintide (Symlin). Pramlintide is an injectable medication used to treat diabetes. It is given as a shot at the same time that a diabetic would take a shot of insulin. The problem is that pramlintide has to be taken as a separate shot from insulin. So diabetics who take pramlintide end up taking seven or more shots each day. Most endocrinologists consider this a "niche" drug and seldom prescribe it.

The advantage of pramlintide is that it has weight loss as a side effect. It also reduces the total amount of insulin a person with diabetes has to take. It can have nausea as a side effect, and some have suggested that it's the nausea that is responsible for the weight loss.

But many people who don't have nausea still lose weight on it. Pramlintide reduces appetite and slows the release of food from the stomach. This slows the rate at which food enters the intestines and increases the feeling of being full.

Pramlintide is FDA approved for the treatment of diabetes and for use in combination with insulin only. But recent research on pramlintide used in combination with synthetic leptin has shown some exciting results in the field of weight loss.

In a research abstract presented at the 2006 meeting of the American Diabetes Association, scientists released the results of a study on the effects of leptin and amylin given to obese rats with leptin resistance. The results were astounding. They showed that when amylin and leptin are combined, it resulted in decreased food intake and decreased body weight at rates much greater than when either leptin or amylin was given alone. For the first time, researchers were able to demonstrate that it was possible to overcome leptin resistance with synthetic leptin.

In the past, leptin injections have been given to humans with leptin resistance, but the results have been disappointing. This breakthrough research on rats has given new hope of finding a way to treat obesity in humans with synthetic leptin and pramlintide combined. For more information on pramlintide, please see Chapter 15.

PART II

METABOLIC HORMONES

5

INSULIN RESISTANCE AND METABOLIC SYNDROME

Insulin Resistance Means Leptin Resistance

An unavoidable consequence of weight gain is insulin resistance. With insulin resistance comes leptin resistance. Leptin resistance and insulin resistance always occur together. When you gain weight, levels of both insulin and leptin rise as your body tries to overcome the resistance. The best treatments for insulin resistance concentrate on improving the way the insulin receptor functions.

Many factors contribute to the development of insulin resistance. The more factors you have, the more severe the insulin resistance. Factors include:

- Aging
- Chronic pain
- Fat in the belly (visceral fat)
- Genetics
- Infection or illness
- Inflammation
- Kidney problems
- Leptin resistance
- Liver problems
- Low potassium levels
- Menopause
- Mental illness
- Obesity or being overweight
- Physical inactivity
- Poor diet
- Pregnancy
- Puberty
- Smoking
- Stress

CAUSES OF INSULIN RESISTANCE

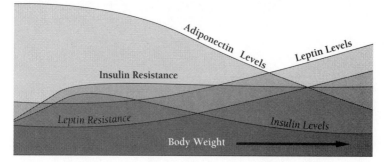

As you gain weight you start to develop insulin and leptin resistance. This leads to fat cell dysfunction and pancreatic burnout. As the pancreatic function declines, there is lower insulin production. When insulin supply cannot keep up with demand, blood sugar rises leading to prediabetes and ultimately diabetes.

Insulin resistance and leptin resistance are intimately linked. The two go hand in hand. It's just like other parts of the body: when one system goes awry, others follow. Insulin resistance makes fat cells produce more TNF-α, a toxic hormone that causes inflammation. Excess fat, especially in the belly, causes insulin resistance, elevated blood sugar, dyslipidemia, and high blood pressure, as well as increased blood clotting and increased inflammation.

Although insulin resistance is the most common hormone problem in the world today, most people don't even know they have it. It is the key factor in conditions like type 2 diabetes, the Metabolic Syndrome, obesity, Polycystic Ovary Syndrome (PCOS), high blood pressure, and cardiovascular disease. But since insulin resistance and leptin resistance go hand in hand, treatments that help the one will naturally help the other, and vice versa. In fact most fat cell hormones are linked to insulin resistance. Adiponectin levels go down as insulin resistance goes up. Diabetes medications that improve insulin resistance can also cause dramatic improvements of adiponectin levels.

INSULIN RESISTANCE AND LEPTIN RESISTANCE—
LINKS THROUGH THE FAT CELL

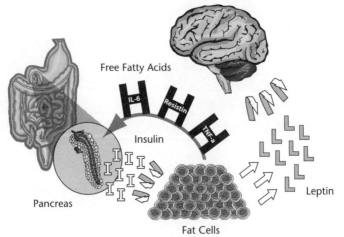

Leptin resistance and insulin resistance go hand in hand. The two conditions per-
petuate each other, becoming a vicious cycle. Insulin resistance means that the fat
cell is blind to the effects of insulin. The fat cell responds by producing excess free
fatty acids, which cause a condition called lipotoxicity that worsens insulin resistance.
Elevated insulin levels also stimulate the production of excess fat in the abdomen, in
muscles, and inside organs. This excess fat produces toxic hormones like TNF-α, IL-
6, resistin, and others. These hormones cause both leptin resistance and insulin
resistance. The cycle continues— perpetuating weight gain and low metabolism.

Insulin resistance is just like other forms of hormone resistance: the receptor for the hormone is dysfunctional. People with
insulin resistance make more insulin to overcome the resistance,
but the consequence is increased appetite and weight gain.
Increased insulin levels cause food to be stored as fat instead of
being burned as energy.

The hallmark of insulin resistance is increased visceral fat. This
is the toxic fat that accumulates in the belly and is a major risk factor for heart attacks and strokes. People with increased fat in the
belly are said to have an apple shape, when compared to those who
have more fat in the hips and legs, called a pear shape. Please see
Chapter 2 for more information on visceral fat.

Free Fatty Acids & Lipotoxicity: The Toxic Effect of Fat

Insulin resistance makes fat cells dysfunctional in many ways. The normal biological processes that regulate energy balance and metabolism go out of whack. Insulin resistance makes fat cells leak their contents, known as free fatty acids, into the circulation. It's normal to have some free fatty acids in your blood. Indeed, free fatty acids form the building blocks for many important chemicals in your body. But if free fatty acid levels go too high, problems occur.

Free fatty acids have a toxic effect on the insulin receptor. This is called lipotoxicity, which means the toxic effect of fat. The free fatty acids intensify insulin resistance, in a vicious cycle. Insulin resistance increases levels of free fatty acid, which worsen insulin resistance. The result: very high free fatty acid levels.

Excess free fatty acids have another effect on the fat cell: they blunt its ability to make leptin. And this is just the time when the brain needs as much leptin as it can get. Insulin resistance and leptin resistance flare but the body can't compensate, because all those extra free fatty acids are poisoning the fat cell.

Metabolic Syndrome

Metabolic Syndrome is a constellation of medical problems that are part of the insulin resistance syndrome. It gives sufferers an increased risk for cardiovascular disease, diabetes, and premature death. Some 60 million Americans have Metabolic Syndrome. The criteria for Metabolic Syndrome are if you have three or more of the following:

- **Elevated blood sugar:** Fasting blood glucose of 100 mg/dL or above.
- **Increased belly fat:** Waist circumference 35 inches or greater for women, 40 inches or greater for men.
- **Elevated blood pressure:** Blood pressure 130/85 mmHg or higher.

- **High triglycerides:** Fasting triglyceride level 150 mg/dL or above.
- **Decreased good cholesterol:** HDL cholesterol 50 mg/dL or less in women, 40 mg/dL or less in men.

For more information, you should read my book *Overcoming Metabolic Syndrome.* The book is a guide to help you better understand and overcome this complex disorder.

DIAGNOSTIC CRITERIA FOR METABOLIC SYNDROME
(3 or more of the following)
• Fasting Blood Glucose > 100 mg/dL
• Waist Circumference > 35 inches in women or > 40 inches in men
• Blood Pressure > 130/85 mmHg
• Fasting Triglycerides > 150 mg/dL
• HDL Cholesterol < 50 mg/dL in women or < 40 mg/dL in men

Carbohydrate Cravings and Hypoglycemia

Insulin resistance and leptin resistance can lead to problems with how the body perceives sugars and starches it receives by way of food. This can lead to symptoms commonly referred to as carbohydrate cravings, or "carb" cravings. Typical symptoms of carbohydrate cravings include feeling tired or sleepy in the afternoon, feeling hungry or having heart palpitations two or three hours after meals, after feeling anxious gaining a feeling of calmness by eating high-carb foods. Carbohydrate cravings are linked to leptin, insulin, and serotonin. Some research has also linked carbohydrate cravings to excessive use of artificial sweeteners (for more information on this, please see Chapter 14). The Leptin Boost Diet will help you eliminate carbohydrate cravings for good.

Hypoglycemia is a complex problem caused by an exaggerated response of insulin to a high sugar or high carbohydrate meal.

MEDICAL COMPLICATIONS OF INSULIN RESISTANCE

Insulin resistance is associated with many medical complications. Improving leptin resistance will improve insulin resistance and will improve all their complications at the same time. When you balance leptin and insulin, you decrease your risk of these problems:

Acanthosis nigricans
Anxiety
Blood clots
Cancer
Cardiovascular disease
Deep vein thrombosis
Depression
Diabetes
Fatigue
Fatty liver disease
Gallstones
Gout
Heart disease
High blood pressure
   (hypertension)
High CRP levels

High LDL (small, dense variety)
   cholesterol
High triglycerides
High uric acid levels
Insomnia
Kidney disease
Low HDL (good) cholesterol
Male hypogonadism
Obstructive sleep apnea
Polycystic Ovary Syndrome (PCOS)
Pregnancy complications
Protein in the urine
Psychiatric problems
Skin problems
Skin tags
Strokes

When someone with insulin resistance eats a meal that is high in sugar or processed carbohydrates, the pancreas can overreact and pump out too much insulin. The result is a rapid lowering of blood sugar, causing symptoms like rapid heart beat, shakiness, dizziness, sweating, or blurred vision. These hypoglycemic symptoms usually come on within a few minutes to a few hours after eating the offending food. The Leptin Boost Diet is great for people with hypoglycemia and will eliminate the symptoms completely for most people. A word of warning, though: in rare cases hypoglycemia is caused by a tumor of the pancreas (known as an *insulinoma*) that pumps out too much insulin. For this reason, if you have any symptoms of hypoglycemia, you should see your physician. Symptoms may include:

- Anxiety
- Blurred vision
- Carb cravings
- Confusion
- Dizziness
- Fatigue
- Heart pounding

- Hunger
- Nervousness
- Rapid heartbeat
- Shakiness
- Sweating
- Tremor

Candida

I have seen many patients who think they have insulin resistance, leptin resistance, or other problems caused by systemic candida infection. Many alternative or natural doctors make claims that candida causes many medical problems, including diabetes, carbohydrate cravings, irritable bowel syndrome, fibromyalgia, asthma, lupus, chronic fatigue syndrome, multiple sclerosis, autism, eczema, psoriasis, scleroderma, arthritis, attention deficit disorder (ADD), headaches, and food allergies. Unfortunately, I have seen patients who have been inappropriately prescribed antifungal medications to fight systemic candida infection.

Experts all agree that candida has nothing to do with these conditions. All humans have candida in our digestive tract; it's part of a healthy body. Severe medical problems, like AIDS and diabetes, can lead to infections with candida, but these are mostly vaginal yeast infections or mouth infections (known as thrush). In one condition known as systemic candidiasis, candida infects the whole body. It is only seen in patients who have severe immune system problems and is a very severe illness producing extremely high fevers. Candida infections can be a real medical problem in people with immune problems. Most people who have been told they have systemic candida infection and that it is a cause of their chronic problems are better served by seeking a second opinion from a more legitimate practitioner.

6

CORTISOL AND THE ADRENAL GLAND

Leptin Is the Link Between Cortisol and Your Weight

Leptin, stress, and cortisol are closely linked. Cortisol is a stress hormone that, when produced in excessive amounts, causes leptin resistance and weight gain. Excess cortisol in one's system leads to slower metabolism, muscle loss, and fat accumulation in unhealthy parts of the body. The body can create yet another vicious circle: too much cortisol will make you gain weight.

Being overweight makes you have leptin resistance, but that's not the only hormone that goes out of whack. Excess weight tells your adrenal glands to produce even more cortisol. Cortisol regulates body fat and its distribution. Excess cortisol worsens both leptin resistance and insulin resistance. To have hormonal balance, your cortisol and leptin must be balanced.

Cortisol and leptin are intimately linked. If one goes out of balance, the other will follow. High cortisol levels cause leptin resistance (along with insulin resistance). This leads to higher cortisol and more leptin resistance. Low leptin levels raise cortisol levels, which cause insulin resistance, so that the small amount of leptin that is still present works less efficiently. One more vicious cycle: leptin and cortisol problems compound each other, worsening the situation.

Many people who are overweight—most notably, those with fat in the belly, a round face, and high blood sugar or high blood pressure—have elevated cortisol levels. Since cortisol makes you gain weight, just being overweight makes you have too much cortisol. The cycle goes around and around.

It's that excess fat in the belly that throws everything off. Too much fat produces hormonal imbalance, leptin resistance, and cortisol excess. Those toxic fat cell hormones, *adipokines*, stimulate the adrenal gland to pump out more cortisol. The result: more cortisol, more fat, and more toxic hormones. Here comes that vicious cycle again. Symptoms of excess cortisol are:

- Acne
- Anxiety
- Broken bones
- Bruising
- Colds/flu
- Decreased sex drive
- Depression
- Facial hair growth (in women)
- Fat in the belly
- Fatigue
- Heartburn or reflux
- High blood pressure
- High blood sugar
- High cholesterol
- High triglycerides
- Increased appetite
- Infections
- Insomnia
- Menstrual cycle problems
- Mood swings
- Muscle weakness
- Osteoporosis or osteopenia
- Poor concentration
- Poor memory
- Red face
- Round face
- Slow metabolism
- Stomach ulcers
- Stretch marks
- Thin arms and legs
- Thin skin
- Upset stomach
- Weakness
- Weight gain

Stress, Cortisol, and Your Weight

Stress causes hormonal imbalance in so many ways. Stress slows one's metabolism and leads to weight gain. One of the main effects of stress is to increase cortisol levels. Any type of stress can increase your cortisol—work stress, family stress, stress from depression or anxiety, even the stress of poor health. One of the more serious forms of stress on the body is excess weight, which leads to chronically elevated cortisol levels. If you don't get enough sleep, or enough good-quality sleep, you can also have increased cortisol levels. But when you lose weight and eliminate or reduce stress in your life, cortisol levels go down.

STRESS, FAT CELL, BRAIN, AND ADRENAL GLAND ARE LINKED THROUGH LEPTIN AND CORTISOL

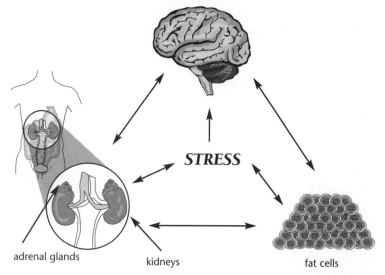

adrenal glands   kidneys   fat cells

Leptin and cortisol provide an important link between fat cells, the adrenal gland, and the brain. Increased stress raises cortisol levels, which increases leptin resistance.

Increased cortisol causes weight gain by increasing the amount of unhealthy fat in your body. It causes the same increases in visceral fat that we see with leptin resistance and insulin resistance. If you have increased visceral fat, it is likely that you have problems with all three hormones.

Cushing's Syndrome

A severe form of cortisol excess, Cushing's Syndrome is caused by a tumor in the pituitary gland or in the adrenal gland. The main treatment for Cushing's Syndrome is surgical removal of the offending gland. I have seen many patients who have been told time and time again that they are overweight because they eat too much, only to discover that their real problem was a tumor. The testing for Cushing's Syndrome can be tricky. In fact, there is no perfect test. Early diagnosis and treatment is critical for this potentially devastating hormonal disorder. Some warning signs are:

- Abnormal menstrual cycle
- Acne
- Anxiety
- Depression
- Easy bruising
- Excessive weight gain
- Facial hair growth (in women)
- Fat on the back of the neck
- Fat over the collar bones
- Frequent infections
- High blood pressure
- High blood sugar
- Low testosterone (in men)
- Male pattern balding (in women)
- Muscle weakness
- Rapid weight gain
- Round face
- Stretch marks
- Thin skin

For more information on Cushing's Syndrome please see my book, *Hormonal Balance: Understanding Hormones, Weight, and Your Metabolism.*

Cortisol, Leptin, and Your Brain

Leptin and cortisol are linked through connections in the hunger centers of the brain—the hypothalamus. Corticotropin-releasing hormone (CRH) is a hormone produced by the hypothalamus, the same region where leptin takes its effect. CRH works by telling the pituitary gland to make a hormone that ultimately stimulates the adrenal gland to ramp up cortisol production. CRH is influenced by the brain hormone neuropeptide Y (NPY). For more information on NPY, please see Chapter 3. Neuropeptide Y is a potent stimulator of appetite and cravings. Under normal circumstances, leptin works to keep neuropeptide levels down. If you have leptin resistance or leptin deficiency, NPY levels go up.

Increased NPY hikes the production of a corticotropin-releasing hormone, which stimulates the pituitary gland to tell the adrenal gland to make more cortisol.

THE RELATIONSHIP BETWEEN CORTISOL, LEPTIN, AND THE BRAIN

CRH is the critical link between leptin and cortisol. Leptin works in the brain to decrease levels of the hunger hormone NPY. If you have leptin resistance or insulin resistance, NPY levels go up, increasing production of the hormone CRH, which ultimately leads to increased cortisol levels. These, in turn, cause weight gain and leptin resistance.

Cortisol-Lowering Supplements

Many nutritional supplements are being promoted with the promise that they will lower your cortisol levels and help you lose weight. For the most part, these supplements are a scam. They contain ingredients like green tea extract, bitter orange peel, ginseng, passionflower, magnolia bark, citrus aurantium, beta-sitoserol, chromium, jujuba fruit, and vanadyl sulfate. The Federal Trade Commission has charged certain marketers with claiming, falsely, that their products can cause weight loss and reduce the risk of, or even prevent, serious health conditions. The manufacturer paid about $4.5 million in a settlement. Despite this, many such products remain on the market. I recommend avoiding them entirely.

7

THYROID HORMONE

Leptin Resistance
Causes Thyroid Dysfunction

It's estimated that from 20 to 30 million Americans have some form of thyroid disease. And when your thyroid is out of balance, you are likely to have leptin problems. Thyroid problems present patients with a wide variety of medical complaints. Each person is affected differently: you may have one, two, or many symptoms. Any or all of the body's organ systems may be influenced by changes in the thyroid. When weight problems begin, many people suspect that the thyroid gland may be at fault. The thyroid is a potent regulator of appetite and body weight that interacts with leptin to maintain hormonal balance.

Leptin and thyroid hormone interact in a push-and-pull manner. If there's a problem with leptin, the thyroid suffers, and vice versa. Thyroid-stimulating hormone (TSH) and leptin follow similar diurnal hormonal fluxes, peaking in the middle of the night. Signals for thyroid hormone production begin in the hypothalamus—the very same area where leptin has its effect. The hypothalamus produces a hormone that goes to the pituitary gland, called TRH, or thyrotropin-releasing hormone. Neurons that make TRH have receptors for leptin and are highly responsive to the leptin in your body. The pituitary gland reacts to TRH by releasing another hormone, TSH, or thyroid-stimulating hormone. TSH travels through the bloodstream to the thyroid gland. TSH tells to the thyroid gland to produce thyroid hormones. The hypothalamus is responsible for coordinating with leptin and other signals to keep the level of thyroid hormones constant.

Leptin has a major effect on the hypothalamus and pituitary gland and the way they regulate the thyroid gland. Leptin is required for proper function of the brain and thyroid gland. When there is a problem with leptin, it will be accompanied by a thyroid problem. Low leptin levels and leptin resistance will do the same thing to the thyroid—slowing brain signals, and ultimately reducing thyroid hormone levels.

Sick Euthyroid Syndrome is a term used to describe the thyroid's response to extreme illness. It's thought of as being an adaptive response. During times of extreme stress, such as during starvation, the brain shuts down thyroid function to slow metabolism and preserve body fat. Leptin is the primary mediator in this process. It all goes back to leptin's duty to preserve body fat during starvation. The problem is that *any* kind of stress can induce this adaptive response, so even if you are not starving, your brain will think you are and will work (through leptin) to lower thyroid function.

When you have Sick Euthyroid Syndrome, the thyroid is perfectly fine, but it doesn't do much because it is trying to preserve a sick body. This is a hard condition to diagnose, because thyroid tests typically come out normal. Some people try to take thyroid hormone medications to treat Sick Euthyroid Syndrome. These medications do not work in this situation. The best treatment is to alleviate the stress on the body, whereupon your leptin–thyroid balance will return naturally.

If the stress on your body is obesity, then leptin resistance is the mediator behind your thyroid problems. As you lose weight, your leptin resistance will improve and your thyroid will function more efficiently.

Hypothyroidism

As many as 25 million Americans suffer from some form of thyroid disease. The most common type of thyroid problem is low levels of thyroid hormone, known as hypothyroidism. The chief symptoms of hypothyroidism are the same as those observed in leptin resistance—slow metabolism, fatigue, and weight gain. When thyroid hormone levels are low, the body's entire hormonal system goes out of balance.

The initial symptoms of hypothyroidism are usually mild and do not concentrate in a specific part of the body. Symptoms may be disregarded or attributed to other causes, such as fibromyalgia, menopause, depression, old age, or life stress. As thyroid levels go lower, the symptoms become more severe. Many people with thyroid problems don't get diagnosed because they attribute their symptoms to those of normal aging. They might experience a little weight gain, feel unusually tired, or have some constipation. And many of the symptoms of hypothyroidism are, in fact, the same those of as normal aging. But if you have any of the following symptoms, it's easy to get tested:

- Allergies
- Constipation
- Decreased sweating
- Depression
- Drowsiness
- Dry skin
- Enlarged thyroid gland
- Fatigue
- Feeling cold
- Gruff voice
- Hair loss
- High cholesterol
- Hoarse voice
- Joint aches
- Memory loss
- Menopausal symptoms
- Menstrual cycle problems
- Muscle aches
- Pale skin
- Poor concentration
- Premature aging
- Slow heartbeat
- Slow metabolism
- Slow reflexes
- Snoring
- Stuffy nose
- Weight gain

For more information on thyroid problems, including details on testing and treatment, please read my book, *A Simple Guide to Thyroid Disorders: From Diagnosis to Treatment* (Addicus Books, 2004).

8

ANDROGENS

Androgen Balance Is Critical for Leptin Balance

Male hormones, also known as androgens, are closely linked to leptin and adiponectin. Even though they are called "male" hormones, both men and women have androgens. In men, low androgens are a major cause of leptin problems, but in women high androgens cause leptin resistance and insulin resistance. As with all your hormones, too much or too little can cause problems—hormonal balance is extremely important. For your leptin to work properly, your androgens must be balanced.

Leptin and testosterone have a push-pull relationship. Low leptin and leptin resistance cause low testosterone and low sperm counts. Low testosterone leads to leptin resistance. Once more, the vicious cycle. The two compound each other, slowing metabolism and leading to fatigue and weight gain.

Weight loss benefits the body in a great many ways. Testosterone balance is no exception. In men, weight loss will raise testosterone, while in women, weight loss causes testosterone to go down. These changes are beneficial for achieving hormonal balance and will help you achieve a proper body fat distribution, reducing fat in the middle and increasing metabolism. When your testosterone is balanced, leptin and adiponectin work more efficiently, raising metabolism and lowering appetite.

Androgen hormones, also known as anabolic steroids, get their name from the fact that they promote muscle growth. Androgens are specialized hormones that work by turning on genes that make muscles grow. They help your muscles become stronger—both physically *and* metabolically. Testosterone is the most well known androgen hormone and is the most important androgen when it comes to leptin balance.

The amount of muscle you have is perhaps the most important indicator of your metabolism. Muscle is highly active tissue that needs lots of fuel to keep going. Muscle needs sugar and fat, so it pulls it out of the bloodstream to convert it into energy. The more muscle you have, the more calories you burn, the higher your metabolism, and the higher your energy level will be.

Early leptin research found that the *obese* leptin-deficient mouse had very low testosterone levels. When these mice are given leptin, testosterone levels return to normal. Leptin works to stimulate the hypothalamus and pituitary gland to produce brain hormones necessary for the production of testosterone. Testosterone has a reciprocal effect on leptin. Low testosterone will cause leptin resistance. Low testosterone also leads to low levels of the beneficial fat hormone adiponectin and elevated levels of toxic fat hormones like resistin, TNF-α, and IL-6. These hormones, in turn, inhibit the production of testosterone.

Leptin is intimately connected to testosterone, is needed for normal testosterone production, and is responsible for many hormonal changes that occur in periods of stress or starvation. Leptin, body fat, and reproduction are all interconnected. Studies have shown that men who are malnourished have very low testosterone levels. This normal response of the body is to adapt to by lowering metabolism and shifting energy into survival mode and away from reproductive mode. The stress from starvation causes leptin levels to drop. When leptin levels fall, testosterone falls as well. When you lose weight, you should do it in a way that will improve leptin resistance and not make leptin fall. The Leptin Boost Diet will help you lose weight without impeding your body's ability to make leptin and testosterone.

It is thought that leptin is one of the critical mediators responsible for the low testosterone levels in obese men. This condition, known as obesity-induced hypogonadism, is very common and frequently not diagnosed. Leptin resistance means that the brain is blind to the effects of leptin. As are the hypothalamus and pituitary gland. Once this happens, the production of brain hormones falls and testosterone follows.

THE RELATIONSHIP BETWEEN LEPTIN AND TESTOSTERONE IN MEN

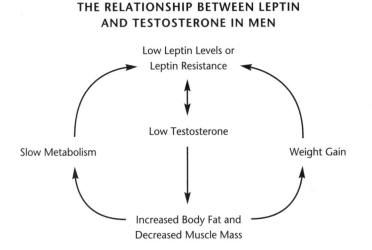

Proper leptin levels are required for adequate testosterone production. If leptin levels drop, or there is leptin resistance, testosterone production will fall. Similarly, if testosterone production drops, leptin levels will decline. Low testosterone leads to decreased muscle mass, decreased metabolism, and weight gain. This, in turn, increases leptin resistance…and the cycle continues.

Hypogonadism

When men have low testosterone (also known as hypogonadism, male menopause, or "low T"), leptin goes out of balance. Low testosterone results in an increase of belly fat, known as visceral fat. This toxic fat is one of the major causes of leptin resistance and low adiponectin levels. Muscles become smaller and get infiltrated with fat. The fat that penetrates muscles, known as intramuscular fat, is just like the metabolically evil fat that's found in the belly. This increases the risk of heart attacks, strokes, and diabetes. Testosterone is vital for leptin balance because, without it, there's too much bad fat around and there are more toxic fat hormones like TNF-α, IL-6, and resistin. These hormones slow metabolism and worsen both leptin and insulin resistance. Leptin resistance lowers testosterone even further, and so the cycle continues.

Obese men commonly have very low testosterone, caused by leptin resistance. It is known as *central hypogonadism*, because the cause is a deficiency of the hormones produced by the central nervous system that cause the testicles to make testosterone. Under normal circumstances, leptin works in the brain—at the hypothalamus and pituitary gland—to stimulate production of hormones known as gonadotropins. These hormones—gonadotropin-releasing hormone (GnRH), lutenizing hormone (LH), and follicle-stimulating hormone (FSH)—stimulate the testicles to produce testosterone. If the body lacks sufficient leptin, or has leptin resistance, there will be problems with achieving proper levels of GnRH, LH, FSH, and ultimately testosterone. It's all part of nature's balance. When there's leptin resistance, the brain thinks the body is starving because it's blind to leptin. Part of its defense mechanism is to shut down all bodily functions not critical for survival.

If you have central hypogonadism, your blood tests may show normal LH and FSH levels. Normal LH and FSH levels in the setting of low testosterone levels are the typical pattern seen in men with hypogonadism caused by leptin resistance.

Obesity-induced hypogonadism is a very common cause of low testosterone in men. Treatment not only improves the symptoms of hypogonadism but improves leptin resistance and helps with weight loss as well. In my clinical practice, I find that many men with untreated low testosterone make dramatic improvements once they go on testosterone replacement therapy (TRT). Low testosterone is associated with decreased muscle size and strength, increased body fat, depression, diminished sense of well-being, fatigue, low sex drive, erectile dysfunction, osteoporosis, and increased risk for heart disease. Low testosterone can occur slowly or abruptly. But at whatever rate it occurs, if you have these symptoms, you should see your physician:

- Anxiety
- Decreased performance in sports
- Depression
- Erectile dysfunction
- Excessive sweating
- Fatigue
- Flushing
- Hot flashes
- Increased body fat
- Insomnia
- Low sex drive
- Muscle weakness
- Poor attention span
- Poor memory
- Premature aging
- Weight gain

Leptin and Puberty in Boys

In addition to its effects on appetite and weight, leptin has potent effects on the male reproductive system. Leptin is responsible for signaling the brain to begin the hormonal changes of puberty. It is thought that puberty occurs when the body accumulates enough body fat. Leptin is the key signal for this process. This explains why boys who are overweight tend to go through puberty earlier than their normal-weight peers. Unfortunately, an earlier-than-normal puberty means you stop growing earlier and your overall height is less than it otherwise would be. With the epidemic of extreme obesity in adolescent boys, we are starting to see a new phenomenon. Leptin resistance is making these boys have a late puberty, increasing their overall height. I have seen many 15- and 16-year-old boys who are over six feet tall and weigh well over 300 pounds!

Male Hormones in Women

High testosterone levels in women have the same effect on leptin and adiponectin as does low testosterone in men. High androgens, also known as *hyperandrogenism,* cause leptin resistance, low adiponectin levels, and insulin resistance. There's a direct correlation to between a woman's weight and her androgen levels. The heavier she is, the higher her male hormone levels will be.

Testosterone is an important androgen in women. It's made by the ovaries. Unlike men, in whom testosterone is the main hormone, two other important androgen hormones also help regulate female androgen balance. The first, androstenedione, is a weaker androgen produced by the ovary. The second, DHEA-S, is a male hormone made by the adrenal gland.

Symptoms of androgen excess include weight gain, especially around the middle; menstrual cycle problems (irregular cycles, skipped cycles, or no cycle; cramping); facial hair growth; hair loss; acne; infertility; high blood pressure; and deepening of the voice.

SYMPTOMS OF POLYCYSTIC OVARY SYNDROME

Abnormal menstrual cycles	Family history of diabetes
Acanthosis nigricans	Hair loss
Anxiety	Infertility
Depression	Poor body image
Excess fat in the belly	Skin tags
Excessive menstrual cramps	Stretch marks
Facial hair growth	Weight gain

Diagnostic criteria for PCOS

Any 2 of the following:

- Menstrual cycle problems (missed cycles, irregular cycles, heavy cycles, frequent cycles, light cycles, painful cycles)
- Hyperandrogenism (skin problems—adult acne, facial hair growth, or elevated androgen blood tests)
- Polycystic ovaries (on ultrasound)

Other disorders causing hyperandrogenism must also be excluded

Androgen excess, or hyperandrogenism, can be caused by overactive ovaries or overactive adrenal glands. Polycystic Ovary Syndrome (PCOS) is the most common cause of androgen excess in women. PCOS is closely linked to insulin resistance and leptin resistance, both of which cause a woman's ovaries and adrenal glands to produce excess male hormones. When you lose weight, leptin resistance and insulin resistance improves, adiponectin levels go up, and the symptoms of PCOS improve. The Leptin Boost Diet and the treatment of leptin problems will also improve symptoms of androgen excess.

9

FEMALE HORMONES

Female Hormones and Leptin

Leptin and reproductive function are closely linked through female hormones. This connection is the body's way of telling the brain that a woman's nutritional status is adequate for puberty and childbearing. The more fat a woman has, the higher her leptin. When leptin goes up, the body ramps up estrogen production. Fat cells make an enzyme called *aromatase*, which converts male hormones into estrogen. So as you gain weight, fat cells have a greater influence on your balance of male and female hormones.

Estrogen is responsible for the female body shape—excess fat goes to the hips and buttocks. It puts on the fat that makes the healthy fat cell hormones like leptin and adiponectin. When a woman goes through menopause and has lower estrogen levels, this healthy fat is shifted to the belly. The fat cells become visceral adipocytes, the "bad boys" of fat cell endocrinology—producing toxic fat cell hormones like resistin, TNF-α, and IL-6.

Women with anorexia stop having their menstrual cycle because of leptin. When body fat stores drop, leptin levels also drop and the brain responds by shutting down the production of brain hormones needed for female hormone balance—gonadotropin-releasing hormone (GnRH), lutenizing hormone (LH), and follicle-stimulating hormone (FSH). These hormones coordinate the menstrual cycle and the production of estrogen and progesterone. When leptin goes low, or there's leptin resistance, female hormones go out of balance.

Estrogen is closely tied to the fat cell. Fat cells contain the enzyme aromatase, which converts androgens to estrogens, primarily estrone. Estrone is an unhealthy form of estrogen that causes leptin resistance and insulin resistance. Female hormonal balance means having low estrone levels and higher levels of a healthy estrogen—estradiol.

Estradiol is the best type of estrogen. Healthy young women have high levels of it. Lower estradiol levels will cause leptin resistance. This has advocated some to recommend estrogen-replacement therapy in menopausal women as a way of improving leptin resistance. Estrogen replacement therapy, or ERT, when taken in the proper dosage and form, does in fact improve leptin resistance and body fat distribution. Hormone replacement therapy, or HRT, is controversial, however. Estrogen has diverse effects and can have both risks and benefits. Estrogen replacement therapy has side effects such as blood clots, heart attacks, strokes, and an increased risk for breast cancer. If you are considering HRT, you should discuss your individual risks and benefits with your physician.

Leptin and Puberty in Girls

Leptin is a key regulator of puberty and sexual development in girls. People with a mutation of the leptin gene—or leptin deficiency—not only have severe obesity but also don't go into puberty. Weight, body fat, and female hormones are tied together, but how does the brain know when to begin producing the hormones needed for puberty?

Leptin serves as a signal to the brain to give information on the vital quantity of fat reserves that are necessary for proper functioning of the pituitary gland and the hypothalamus. Rising leptin levels stimulate puberty, and normal leptin levels are required to maintain normality in the menstrual cycle and reproductive function.

Declining leptin levels in response to weight loss can result in dysfunction of the pituitary gland and hypothalamus, leading to lower estrogen levels and cessation of the menstrual cycle. This is commonly seen in women as anorexia nervosa, as well as in vigorously exercising athletes.

Adolescent girls experience a large increase in fat just before they start their menstrual cycle. This is nature's way of preparing the body for reproduction. The increased fat makes more leptin, which signals the brain that a girl is ready to become a woman. Normally, a girl will double the amount of fat in her body from the beginning of puberty until the end of it. Once leptin levels are high enough, the brain starts off a cascade of female hormones that ultimately leads to the first menstrual cycle. Boys also gain fat during puberty, but they gain much more muscle during that stage, due to increases in the hormone testosterone. Nevertheless, leptin is also an important regulator of puberty in boys as well. Leptin also stimulates the production of growth hormone. A rise in growth hormone is responsible for the growth spurt seen during puberty. For more on growth hormone, please see Chapter 10.

Girls these days are going through puberty earlier than ever before. Today, a girl's first menstrual cycle typically occurs at about 12½ years old. As recently as 100 years ago, the average age was 14; 200 ago, the average age was 17. Researchers believe that girls are going through puberty earlier, largely due to increased body fat and higher leptin levels.

Leptin, Fertility, Pregnancy, and Menopause

To be fertile, women need a certain amount of fat. Thin women, especially those who are underweight, have a lower fertility than women who are of normal weight or slightly overweight. Leptin serves as a signal to the brain that a woman has adequate fat stores in order to be successful at conceiving and having a healthy pregnancy. If the brain detects that the body is underweight, it will shut down fertility, via leptin. If a woman lacks sufficient body fat, she will not produce the hormones necessary for reproduction. Most women need to have a body mass index of 19 kg/m^2 for her reproductive hormones to function properly, but athletic women who have a very low body fat percentage can experience fertility problems at higher weights. For more on the body mass index, please see Chapter 12. The effect of leptin on fertility is totally reversible. Once a woman gains the minimum amount of body fat, all other things being normal, she will regain normal reproductive function.

Leptin exerts some of its effects directly on the uterus, breast, and placenta, with equivalent influence on pregnancy and breast milk production. Leptin is also responsible for the growth of blood vessels that are needed for development of a fetus. Without leptin, a baby will not grow properly.

Interestingly, menopause has no effect on leptin levels. When a woman goes through menopause, estrogen levels fall, but leptin levels remain constant. Obese menopausal women, however, have much higher leptin levels than lean menopausal women.

Leptin and Your Bones

In Chapter 1, I talked about all the health problems associated with being overweight. There is one health benefit of obesity—stronger bones. It makes sense, because the heavier you are, the stronger your bones need to be. Leptin is a critical regulator of bone health. It's your body's way of telling your bones how much you weigh and how strong the bones must be to keep you standing up straight.

Osteoporosis, or thinning of the bones, is common in menopausal women and is more prevalent in lean than in overweight women. It is now known that leptin is an important hormone responsible for proper bone health. Leptin can inhibit bone formation, and high leptin levels are thought to be a cause of osteoporosis. Leptin-deficient mice and humans not only have increased amounts of fat but also have stronger bones. When leptin is given to individuals with leptin deficiency, not only do they lose weight, they lose bone too. More research is needed in this area, but it is thought that leptin's effect on bones is through a totally different pathway from the one that causes its effect on weight (which is through the brain hormones—neuropeptide Y and POMC). Eventually, medications that specifically block leptin's effect on the bones may be developed as a treatment for osteoporosis.

10

GROWTH HORMONE AND THE PITUITARY GLAND

Leptin and Growth Hormone

Growth hormone and leptin have major influences on each other. Growth hormone is a hormone produced by the pituitary gland whose major function is regulating the amount of muscle and fat in your body. Leptin signals the brain how much fat is in your body. When leptin levels go up, growth hormone also goes up. A burst of leptin during puberty, for example, causes a burst of growth hormone. This rise in growth hormone is responsible for the growth spurt seen during puberty.

As you read further in this book, you'll see that the amount of fat you have in your body is the most important determinant of your metabolism, or metabolic rate. So, growth hormone is a critical determinant of your metabolism. If you have low levels of growth hormone, you will have low metabolism and increased body fat. This will eventually lead to weight gain and even lower growth hormone levels. Low growth hormone will also cause leptin resistance, and (here comes that vicious cycle again) leptin resistance causes lower growth hormone levels.

Growth hormone was once thought of as a hormone that was only important for making children grow. Children with low growth hormone will have a short stature unless they are treated with growth hormone replacement therapy. We now know that growth hormone is an important hormone for adults as well.

Growth hormone (or GH) deficiency can make you gain weight. And studies show that GH replacement helps improve leptin resistance while helping you lose fat and gain muscle.

Low growth hormone levels are also a cause of depression, anxiety, and social isolation. Growth hormone replacement will help improve your mood and gives you more energy, so that you'll feel like exercising.

For those who are GH deficient, growth hormone replacement will decrease the amount of fat in your body and will increase your

GROWTH HORMONE AND LEPTIN

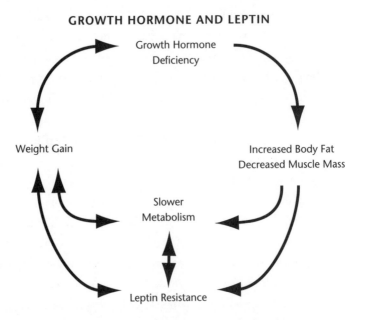

Growth hormone and leptin have major influences on each other. Low growth hormone levels, or growth hormone deficiency, causes increased fat and decreased muscle mass, leading to decreased metabolism and leptin resistance. Leptin resistance further slows metabolism and leads to weight gain. The weight gain makes growth hormone levels decline further, and the cycle continues.

muscle mass. Growth hormone replacement also improves exercise performance, heart function, mood, and your sense of well-being. Growth hormone therapy is, however, not for everyone. Excesses of growth hormone can also cause problems, such as leptin resistance, insulin resistance, diabetes, high blood pressure, arthritis, and swelling.

Growth hormone originally got its name because it makes children grow taller. But in adults it works because it makes muscles grow. Growth hormone and testosterone (please see Chapter 8) have similar effects on your body composition—increasing muscle mass and decreasing fat.

The main function of growth hormone is to direct the liver to make a secondary hormone called insulin-like growth factor-1, or IGF-1 (also known as somatomedin C). IGF-1 is the hormone that does all the work for growth hormone.

Growth Hormone Deficiency and Excess

People with growth hormone deficiency are commonly overweight and have a higher percentage of body fat. GH deficiency causes the same type of central obesity that is seen with leptin resistance, insulin resistance, type 2 diabetes, high cholesterol, and cardiovascular disease. The main cause of growth hormone deficiency has always been thought to be problems with the pituitary gland. New research, however, has found that obesity itself causes growth hormone deficiency as well. Growth hormone replacement for growth hormone deficiency is still a highly controversial topic. Most endocrinologists agree that patients with pituitary disease should be treated with injections of human growth hormone. But most specialists in that field will not treat growth hormone deficiency unless there is evidence of pituitary disease.

On rare occasions, the pituitary gland can become overactive and produce excess growth hormone. This condition, known as *acromegaly*, results in very high growth hormone levels and can cause insulin resistance and leptin resistance. Too much or too little growth hormone can be a problem. The key, as always, is hormonal balance.

Leptin Resistance Causes Growth Hormone Deficiency

Growth hormone deficiency is usually caused by problems with the pituitary gland or the hypothalamus. But there is also a condition called *obesity-related hyposomatotropism*. In this condition, a person's excess weight blocks the production of growth hormone via leptin. This type of growth hormone deficiency is the type that improves with weight loss. Researchers believe that leptin is the major link between obesity and low levels of growth hormone.

SYMPTOMS OF . . .	
. . . Growth Hormone Deficiency	**. . . Growth Hormone Excess**
Decreased exercise capacity	Acanthosis nigricans
Decreased kidney function	Arthritis
Decreased libido	Broadening of the nose
Decreased muscle mass	Carpal tunnel syndrome
Depression	Change in appearance
Difficulties with sex life	Deepening of the voice
Difficulty relating to others	Diabetes
Dry skin	Elevated blood pressure
Emotional irritability	Elevated blood sugar
Fatigue	Elevated cholesterol
Heart disease	Enlarged tongue
High LDL (bad) cholesterol	Furrowing of the forehead
Increased body fat	Growth of hands and feet
Insomnia	Heart disease
Lack of a sense of well-being	Increased spaces between the teeth
Lack of energy	Protrusion of the jaw
Loss of zest for life	Skin tags
Low HDL (good) cholesterol	Thickened brow
Memory problems	Weight gain
Muscle weakness	
Osteopenia	
Osteoporosis	
Poor general health	
Premature aging	
Social isolation	
Thin skin	
Weight gain	
Wrinkling skin	

PART III

LOSING WEIGHT THROUGH LEPTIN

11

DIAGNOSING LEPTIN PROBLEMS

The symptoms of leptin resistance can run from vague to nonexistent. Being overweight is enough to suggest that you probably have leptin resistance. Sometimes the only symptom of leptin resistance or low adiponectin is fatigue. Many of my patients have had unexplained fatigue for many years, only to learn it was a result of an imbalance of fat cell hormones.

Other symptoms of leptin and adiponectin problems include insomnia, feeling bloated or tired after dinner, carbohydrate cravings, anxiety, getting tired walking up a flight of stairs, dizziness, frequent urination, or slightly blurred vision. As time goes on, the symptoms may worsen.

As you learned in previous chapters, leptin resistance and insulin resistance go hand in hand. Therefore, symptoms of insulin resistance are one of the best ways to diagnose leptin resistance. Most of the time, if you have one or more physical features, you have a high likelihood of having leptin resistance.

Physical Signs and Symptoms

Excess Body Weight or Unexplained Weight Gain

Unexplained weight gain is one of the more common symptoms of leptin resistance. It is the heart of the cycle of hormone imbalance that sets off the cascade of other problems that make you keep gaining more and more weight. The heavier you are, the more likely you are to have leptin resistance and low adiponectin levels. People with a body mass index of 25–27 kg/m^2 or greater are at the most risk. Please see Chapter 12 for more information on the body mass index.

Excess Fat in the Middle

Weight in the abdominal region (visceral fat) is a major indicator of leptin resistance. Also known as *android obesity* or *central obesity*, it's the fat in the middle that dramatically worsens leptin resistance. People with excess belly fat also have insulin resistance. Men with a waistline of more than 40 inches and women with a waistline of more than 35 inches have central obesity and are at high risk for low adiponectin and leptin resistance.

High Body Fat

Although testing methods for body fat vary, experts agree that increased body fat, especially in the belly, inside the muscles, and in the organs, is a major contributor to leptin resistance and high adiponectin levels. Even if you are not overweight, if you are out of shape and have flabby muscles, you will have hormonal imbalance. People with a high percentage of body fat are at increased risk of cardiovascular disease and diabetes and have a sluggish metabolism associated with fat cell hormone imbalance.

Fatigue

One symptom of leptin resistance and low adiponectin levels is fatigue, caused by the body's shifting into fat storage mode. The food that you consume is stored as fat instead of burned as energy. When you improve your fat cell hormones, you will have more energy. In fact, many of my patients who didn't even think they felt tired will tell me that they feel so much better when they lose weight that they didn't realize how bad they felt to start with.

Insomnia

Poor sleep can be both a cause of leptin resistance as well as a symptom. Like many things in the hormonal world, it becomes a vicious cycle. The worse your sleep, the worse your leptin resistance. To boost leptin, you must get good sleep.

High Blood Pressure

People with blood pressure above 130/85 are at increased risk of having leptin resistance and low adiponectin levels.

Acanthosis Nigricans

This is a skin condition linked to insulin resistance, leptin resistance, and low adiponectin levels. The skin shows a dark skin rash or blackish discoloration around the neck, in the armpits, or in other skin folds. It looks like dirt, but it won't wash off. But as you balance your hormones and lose weight, acanthosis nigricans can disappear.

Skin Tags

Small bits of skin projecting from the surrounding skin, called skin tags, are a common sign of leptin resistance and insulin resistance.

Stretch Marks

The appearance of stretch marks can be a sign of leptin resistance and excess cortisol levels. Deep red or purple stretch marks are of particular concern.

Symptoms of Polycystic Ovary Syndrome (in Women)

Symptoms of PCOS, such as facial hair growth, abnormal menstrual cycle, acne, or fertility problems, are part of leptin resistance and insulin resistance.

Symptoms of Hypogonadism (in Men)

Hypogonadism, or low testosterone, is extremely common in men with leptin problems. Testosterone and leptin have powerful effects on one another, so if one has problems, the other follows. Men can experience many symptoms of low testosterone. The most infamous of these are erectile dysfunction and low sex drive, but these are not the most common. In fact, fatigue, depression, and weight gain are much more common. If you have any of the symptoms of low testosterone, I recommend that you see your physician to be tested.

Getting Your Leptin Tested

Leptin testing is still something that's mostly done on an experimental basis. Blood tests have recently become available for clinical use, but it is not commonly done. The normal range for leptin is 1.2-9.5 ng/mL in men and 4.1-25 ng/mL in women. For most people, it's better to use surrogate markers to make an estimation of your level of leptin resistance.

Blood Sugar Testing

Blood sugar testing is a good way to check for leptin resistance. If your blood sugar is elevated, by even a small amount, you have a high probability of having leptin resistance. The best time to measure your blood sugar is first thing in the morning after a 12-hour fast. This is called a fasting blood sugar measurement. Most experts agree that a fasting blood sugar above 95 mg/dL is highly suspect and an indicator that someone might have leptin resistance. You can measure blood sugar at random times during the day. The oral glucose tolerance test, or OGTT, measures the response of your blood sugar to a glucose drink. The OGTT is a sensitive way of detecting subtle blood sugar problems, also known as prediabetes, which is indicative of leptin resistance.

BLOOD SUGAR TESTING
Fasting Blood Sugar Levels Normal: below 95 mg/dL Impaired Fasting Glucose: 100–125 mg/dL Diabetes: 126 mg/dL and above
Random Blood Sugar Levels Normal: 140 mg/dL or below Prediabetes: 140–199 mg/dL Diabetes: 200 mg/dL and above
Two-hour Stimulated Glucose Levels **(after drinking 75 grams of glucose)** Normal: 140 mg/dL or below Impaired Glucose Tolerance: 140–199 mg/dL Diabetes: 200 mg/dL and above

Hemoglobin A1c

A1c, or hemoglobin A1c, is a test that gives an estimate of your average blood sugar level over the last two to three months. A1c levels above 5.6 percent suggest leptin resistance.

TRANSLATING HEMOGLOBIN A1C AND AVERAGE BLOOD SUGARS	
A1c 4%= Blood Sugar 60 mg/dL	A1c 9%= Blood Sugar 210 mg/dL
A1c 5%= Blood Sugar 90 mg/dL	A1c 10%= Blood Sugar 240 mg/dL
A1c 6%= Blood Sugar 120 mg/dL	A1c 11%= Blood Sugar 270 mg/dL
A1c 7%= Blood Sugar 150 mg/dL	A1c 12%= Blood Sugar 300 mg/dL
A1c 8%= Blood Sugar 180 mg/dL	A1c 13%= Blood Sugar 330 mg/dL

Plasminogen Activator Inhibitor-1 (PAI-1)

PAI-1 is a fat cell protein that increases blood clotting. The test is now available from many commercial laboratories. Leptin resistance is associated with elevations in PAI-1 levels. PAI-1 elevations are associated with an increased risk of cardiovascular disease.

Homocysteine

In high levels, the substance known as homocysteine will increase your risk of leptin resistance. It's a cause of blood clots and cardiovascular disease, even among people who have normal cholesterol.

C-reactive Protein (CRP)

The CRP test is a measure of inflammation, which is the main cause of leptin resistance. CRP levels will be elevated with any type of inflammation—such as when the body experiences infection, injury, or other stress.

Low risk: Less than 1.0 mg/L

Average risk: 1–3 mg/L

High risk: Greater than 3.0 mg/L

Urine Microalbumin

This test measures very small quantities of protein in the urine. The test is very sensitive and will detect extremely low levels of protein. People with leptin resistance, insulin resistance, diabetes, and high blood pressure all may have high levels of protein in their urine.

Lipid Testing: Cholesterol and Triglycerides

Leptin resistance is linked to high LDL (bad) cholesterol and low HDL (good) cholesterol as well as high triglycerides. Leptin resistance shifts LDL cholesterol to the small, dense, more dangerous type, which further increases atherosclerosis and increases the risk of cardiovascular disease.

Insulin Levels

It's logical to think that high insulin levels are the best way to diagnose insulin resistance. But insulin testing is not usually recom-

CHOLESTEROL AND TRIGLYCERIDE LEVELS

Total Cholesterol Levels

Desirable	less than 200 mg/dL
Borderline high	200–239 mg/dL
High	above 240 mg/dL

HDL (good) Cholesterol Levels

High	60 mg/dL (higher is better)
Normal	40–60 mg/dL
Low	less than 40 mg/dL

LDL (bad) Cholesterol Levels

Ideal	less than 70 mg/dL
Normal	70–100 mg/dL
Borderline high	100–129 mg/dL
High	130–160 mg/dL
Very high	greater than 160 mg/dL

Triglyceride Levels

Ideal	less than 100 mg/dL
Normal	less than 150 mg/dL
High	150–199 mg/dL
Very high	200–499 mg/dL
Extremely high	greater than 500 mg/dL

mended. This is because such testing is still considered inaccurate, and other tests are much better. If insulin is measured, it should be after a 12-hour fast. A fasting insulin level of higher than 10–15 μU/ml increases your risk of insulin and leptin resistance.

Aldosterone and Renin Levels

Aldosterone is a hormone produced by the adrenal glands that causes high blood pressure and low potassium levels. Renin is a hormone produced by the kidney that stimulates the adrenal gland to make aldosterone. If you have high blood pressure, there's about a 10 percent chance that you have problems with renin or aldosterone. If you have high blood pressure and low potassium (or you are taking potassium supplements to keep your potassium level normal), you should be tested. Diagnosis of the aldosterone or renin problems is very important, because the cause can be a tumor either in the adrenal gland, which may need to be removed surgically, or in the arteries going to the kidneys, which may need to be enlarged with a procedure called angioplasty.

Androgen Levels

Measuring androgen levels can be an important clue in diagnosing leptin problems in both men and women. Leptin resistance causes low testosterone in men and can cause high testosterone, as well as high DHEA-S and high androstenedione levels in women. There are many different ways of measuring androgens, each with advantages and disadvantages. For a detailed description of androgen testing, I recommend that you read my book, *Hormonal Balance: Understanding Hormones, Weight, and Your Metabolism.*

COMMONLY PERFORMED ANDROGEN TESTS	
Total Testosterone	Androstenedione
Free Testosterone	LH
Bioavailable Testosterone	FSH
DHEA-S	

Thyroid Testing

Testing for thyroid problems can be straightforward or complicated. Most of the time a simple blood test, known as the TSH test, is adequate to determine if you have a thyroid problem. Thyroid experts agree that the TSH test is the best test when thyroid disease is suspected. TSH levels move in the opposite direction of thyroid hormones, so a high TSH level indicates low thyroid hormone levels. The TSH will start to go up before thyroid hormones drop below the normal range. Because of this, the TSH level is the best marker of early thyroid problems. The normal range for TSH depends on the laboratory, but for most labs the range is quite large. The truth is that most people need their TSH to be toward the lower end of the normal range, and TSH levels that are "high normal" are probably abnormal in most people. Other thyroid tests include ones for thyroxine, triiodothyronine, and thyroid antibodies. For more information on thyroid testing, please read my book, *A Simple Guide to Thyroid Disorders: From Diagnosis to Treatment.*

COMMONLY PERFORMED THYROID TESTS	
TSH	Thyroid Peroxidase Antibody
Free Thyroxine (FT4)	(TPOAb)
Total Thyroxine (TT4)	Thyroglobulin Antibody (TgAb)
Free Triiodothyronine (FT3)	T-3 Resin Uptake (T3RU)
Total Triiodothyronine (TT3)	

Cortisol Testing

It can be difficult to test for cortisol levels. None of the many different ways to measure cortisol is perfect. Cortisol testing is still considered one of the more controversial areas in the field of endocrinology. Frequently, a battery of tests is needed to diagnose a cortisol problem. A test known as the 24-hour urine-free cortisol (UFC) test is one of the better tests to start out with. This is a good way to find out whether you have a cortisol problem; still, many things can cause an increase in the UFC level. Stress of any type will cause increased cortisol levels in the urine. Cortisol levels that are more than four times the normal range indicate a cortisol problem that goes beyond simply stress. An elevated UFC that is less than four times normal is considered to be in a "gray zone" and requires additional testing. The midnight salivary cortisol level is a good way to determine if elevated cortisol levels warrant further evaluation. For more detailed information on cortisol testing, please see my book, *Hormonal Balance: Understanding Hormones, Weight, and Your Metabolism.*

COMMONLY PERFORMED CORTISOL TESTS	
24-hour Urine Free Cortisol (UFC)	Salivary Cortisol Testing
Overnight Dexamethasone	ACTH Level
Suppression Test (DST)	CRH Stimulation Test
Morning Cortisol Level	Adrenal Gland CT Scan
Midnight Cortisol Level	Pituitary Gland MRI Scan

Insulin-like Growth Factor-1

Imbalance of growth hormone, which is produced by the pituitary gland, is a cause of leptin problems. Levels that are too high or too low can cause problems. Insulin-like growth factor-1 (IGF-1) is a hormone produced by the liver that is used as surrogate marker of growth hormone levels. High IGF-1 levels are an indicator of growth hormone excess, known as acromegaly. Low IGF-1 levels can indicate growth hormone deficiency. If you have abnormal IGF-1 levels, you are at risk of having a problem with the pituitary gland or hypothalamus and additional testing should be done. For more information on growth hormone and how it affects leptin, see Chapter 10.

TESTS PERFORMED IN THE EVALUATION OF ABNORMAL IGF-1 LEVELS	
Growth Hormone Stimulation Test (for low levels)	Thyroid Testing
	Male and Female Hormone Testing
Growth Hormone Suppression Test (for high levels)	ACTH level
	Morning Cortisol Level
Prolactin Level	MRI Scan of the Pituitary Gland

Cardiovascular Testing

As you know by now, leptin resistance is a risk factor for cardiovascular disease. I recommend that everyone with leptin resistance be tested to screen for cardiovascular disease. Cardiovascular tests include electrocardiogram (EKG), echocardiogram, treadmill stress test, nuclear cardiac testing, cardiac CT scans, and carotid ultrasound.

Sleep Study (Polysomnography)

Leptin resistance is a major risk factor for a condition called sleep apnea, a condition caused by pressure on the airway from excess fat in the upper chest, neck, and face. The excess weight causes someone to stop breathing for short periods of time during the night. If you have sleep apnea you probably don't even realize that you've stopped breathing. But you might experience symptoms such as severe fatigue and daytime sleepiness, snoring, headaches, memory problems, and restless legs. Sleep apnea is linked to high blood pressure, heart rhythm disturbances, heart attack, stroke, and sudden death. Sleep apnea is diagnosed by using polysomnography, also known as a sleep study.

Liver Ultrasound

Leptin resistance causes the body to store excess fat in the liver. An ultrasound of the liver is a very good way of determining how much fat you have in your liver. Excess fat in the liver is a strong indicator of excess visceral fat. Nonalcoholic fatty liver disease (NAFLD) is a leading cause of cirrhosis of the liver and a major cause of liver disease in the United States.

Pelvic Ultrasound (for Women)

Women with leptin resistance are at high risk of developing cysts in the ovaries, which can be detected with a pelvic ultrasound test. The procedure can also detect a thickened lining of the uterus, known as the endometrium. A thickened endometrium is a risk factor for cancer of the uterus and is commonly seen in women with PCOS and insulin resistance.

12

THE LEPTIN BOOST DIET

What to Do...

If you want to lose weight and keep it off, your hormones must be brought into balance. This means you have to give leptin a boost by making the leptin in your body work more efficiently. Hormonal balance means precisely that—having *all* your hormones balanced. This is because every one of your hormones, in turn, affects all the other hormones. If one hormone is too high or too low, it has downstream effects on your other hormones, and so on, in a ripple effect. Hormonal balance means having achieved the perfect amount of every hormone. It means having a body that's healthy and resilient. Hormonal balance improves virtually every aspect of your life. Your body will be lean and efficient. You won't have excessive hunger or cravings, and your metabolism will work to keep your body at a healthy weight. You will feel more energetic but without stress or anxiety. Your mood will be elevated. You will have deep, restful, rejuvenating sleep every night. You will have a sharp mind. In short, hormonal balance means feeling better and living longer.

Leptin, adiponectin, and other fat cell hormones are a vital part of hormonal balance because they are the hormonal link between your body and your brain. Balancing your fat cell hormones is critical for the proper functioning of your entire body.

TO-DO LIST FOR THE LEPTIN BOOST DIET

- Add an extra vegetable to your meal
- Clean the house
- Do the diet with a friend
- Do two different types of physical activity in the same day
- Drink at least 8 glasses of water every day
- Eat 3 meals and 3 snacks every day
- Eat a minimum of 5 servings of vegetables every day (more is better)
- Eat a minimum of 5 servings of fruit every day (more is better)
- Eat a salad before your meal
- Eat when you feel hungry
- Exercise as often as possible
- Exercise twice in one day
- Find new ways to burn calories (clean the house, plant a garden, shop till you drop)
- Go to the park
- Involve the whole family
- Keep a food diary
- Pick up trash in the neighborhood
- Plan your meals in advance
- Play sports instead of watching them
- Pull weeds
- Reduce stress in your life
- See your doctor
- Take a walk
- Try a fruit smoothie
- Try a new type of exercise
- Try new recipes with healthy foods
- Try the Leptin Boost Diet for just one day
- Wake up early and exercise
- Walk the dog
- Wash the car
- Wash the dog
- Wear a pedometer

The Leptin Boost Diet will help you achieve hormonal balance. This diet works for anyone who wants to lose weight, balance their hormones, or just feel healthier. This is not a fad diet. The Leptin Boost Diet is 100 percent nutritionally sound. The Leptin Boost Diet will help you lose weight and keep it off, because it is designed to eliminate hunger and cravings. Most diets ultimately fail because they are too restrictive. "Don't eat this, don't eat that!" Instead of concentrating on what you should *not* eat, it's better to focus on what you *should* eat. Your goal when on the Leptin Boost Diet is to focus on the "to-do's" instead of the "not to-do's." Adding "to-do" behaviors is an easy way to be successful. The more of these behaviors you add to your daily routine, the more success you'll see. There is only one "not to-do" behavior that I strongly encourage— don't give up!

For the diet to work, you must never be hungry. There is so much food to eat on this diet that your challenge will be to make sure you eat enough food. Many people find it counterintuitive to think that eating more food will help you lose more weight, but this is exactly what I am saying: *eat more to lose more.*

WEIGHT-LOSS ESTIMATES FOR THE LEPTIN BOOST DIET	
Body Weight	4-Week Weight Loss
125–150 pounds	2–3 pounds
150–175 pounds	3–4 pounds
175–200 pounds	4–5 pounds
200–225 pounds	5–6 pounds
225–250 pounds	6–7 pounds
250–275 pounds	7–8 pounds
275–300 pounds	8–9 pounds
300–325 pounds	9–10 pounds

I'm not saying "eat anything you want." But when you eat more of the foods that I recommend, you won't want to eat as much of the unhealthy foods. No food is off limits. In fact, a balanced diet contains many types of foods. In today's society it's next to impossible to have a "perfect" diet. And if you completely eliminate certain foods, you may feel deprived. The key is to eat the "bad" foods in very small portions, and only occasionally. And never forget about eating more and more of the good foods.

THE LEPTIN BOOST DIET

You can lose weight with just about any diet, but 98 percent of people who do so, gain it all back, and even more within three to five years. Most diets eventually fail because of hunger or cravings. The good news is that the Leptin Boost Diet will allow you to lose weight permanently without hunger or cravings.

Weight-Loss Goals

You can achieve tremendous personal satisfaction by setting and achieving goals. And achieving your weight-loss goals is one of the most gratifying by far. You should start your diet with the end in mind. Where do you want to be, in terms of your weight, in one month? Three months? Six months? A year? Twenty years?

You should set realistic weight-loss goals and be prepared to modify them as time goes on. In my experience, most people under-

WEIGHT-LOSS PATTERNS ON THE LEPTIN BOOST DIET

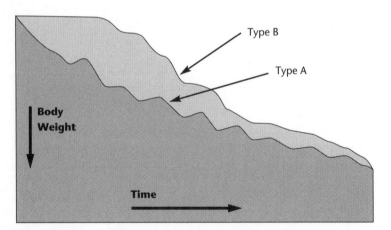

Most people have "Type A" weight loss. This is where there is a large amount of weight loss in the first few weeks, typically 2–8 pounds per week. Weight loss will slow down after this point to 1–2 pounds per week. "Type B" weight loss is where weight remains stable for several weeks before weight loss begins. Individual weight loss amount and rate varies among different people, and these numbers are for rough estimates only. The more closely you follow the diet, the more healthy foods you consume, and the more physical activity you do, the faster the weight-loss will occur.

WEIGHT-LOSS GOALS

Short-Term Goal (1st Month) _____

Mid-Term Goal (3–6 Months) _____

Long-Term Goal (Normal Body Weight) _____

estimate themselves. They want to lose 50 pounds but they don't think they can do it so they set a goal of 20 pounds. Once they lose 20, they feel supercharged and keep losing weight. Next thing they know they've lost 55 pounds! On the Leptin Boost Diet, you can lose all the weight you want to lose—and keep it off forever.

Most people lose about 1 or 2 pounds each week on this diet, but weight loss can vary tremendously and is an individual matter. I've seen people who lose as much as 10 pounds in the first week and others who follow the diet for weeks and only lose a pound or so. The key is to stay on this diet for the long run. Even if you don't see major changes in the first few weeks, eventually you'll notice a major difference. Luckily, however, most people feel better and start losing weight immediately.

Weight loss does not occur in a straight line. Most people will lose more weight in the first few weeks, and then will note that the weight loss slows down a little bit. I recommend weighing yourself only once a week, but you should keep in mind that you will not lose the same amount of weight every week. When I monitor weight loss in my patients, the most important numbers that I follow are the total amount of weight lost and the weight lost over the past four weeks. If you haven't lost much weight in a four-week period, whether at the beginning of the diet or later on, there may be a problem with some of the food you are eating. If this occurs, I recommend increasing the servings of vegetables and fruits and increasing the amount of physical activity to at least one hour every day. This will jump start even the slowest metabolism.

The typical weight-loss pattern is to lose a significant amount of weight, between 2 and 8 pounds per week, in the first couple of

CLASSIFICATION OF WEIGHT BY BMI	
Less than 18.5	Underweight
18.5–25	Normal
25–30	Overweight
30–35	Class I Obesity
35–40	Class II Obesity
Above 40	Class III Obesity
Above 60	Super-Obesity

weeks, then 1 to 2 pounds per week after that. I refer to my patients who lose this way as type A. A few patients, though, have a different weight-loss pattern, which I call type B. They don't lose any weight for a couple of weeks, but then weight loss takes off. In the long run, both type A and type B patients tend to get to their goals in the same amount of time. The problem is that type B patients don't see a lot of results in the beginning and are more likely to get frustrated and give up.

If you don't lose weight in the first couple of weeks, don't give up. You are probably a type B, and will do just fine. Don't lose sight of your goals. Stick with the diet and keep working on getting in more and more fruits, vegetables, and physical activity. In the long run, you'll see big results.

Your long-term goal should be to have a normal body weight. Body weight is assessed using a number called the body mass index, or BMI. The BMI is a calculation based on a person's height and weight.

BMI is calculated by the following formula:

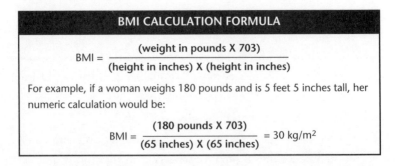

BMI CALCULATION FORMULA

$$BMI = \frac{\text{(weight in pounds X 703)}}{\text{(height in inches) X (height in inches)}}$$

For example, if a woman weighs 180 pounds and is 5 feet 5 inches tall, her numeric calculation would be:

$$BMI = \frac{\text{(180 pounds X 703)}}{\text{(65 inches) X (65 inches)}} = 30 \text{ kg/m}^2$$

It's More Than Just Weight

Hormonal balance means more than simply having a normal body weight. Many people who have a normal weight are quite unhealthy. To be truly healthy, you must have a good balance of muscle and fat in your body. If you have too much body fat, you can have hormonal imbalance even if your weight is normal. The condition has been described as "metabolically obese, normal weight." If you have a high body fat percentage, you'll have leptin resistance and low adiponectin levels. You'll have insulin resistance and low growth hormone levels. If you are a man, your testosterone will be lower; if you are a woman, your testosterone will go up. Fat in the belly, inside the muscles, or in the organs will disrupt hormonal balance and will increase your risk of cardiovascular disease, diabetes, and a multitude of other health problems.

Body fat can be measured in a variety of ways—bioelectrical impedance, skin fold calipers, underwater weighing, CT scans, or DEXA scans, each of which has its advantages and disadvantages. DEXA scans are considered the "gold standard" but are still mostly used for research purposes only. In my medical practice, we use both bioelectrical impedance monitoring and skin fold measurements to assess body fat. Neither one is perfectly accurate, but they give a rough estimate and are a good way of measuring progress. The normal amount of body fat in women is 17 to 27 percent. For men the normal amount is 12 to 24 percent.

Waist circumference is another way to estimate excess body fat. Men with a waist circumference more than 40 inches and women

HORMONAL PROBLEMS ASSOCIATED WITH INCREASED BODY FAT	
Leptin Resistance	Low Growth Hormone
Low Adiponectin	Low Testosterone (in men)
Insulin Resistance	High Testosterone (in women)
High Cortisol	Thyroid Dysfunction

with a waist circumference of more than 35 inches have central obesity and increased amounts of unhealthy body fat.

Most people who are normal weight and have a high percentage of body fat have one thing in common—they are out of shape. People who never exercise, or who exercise less than two hours per week, are the most likely to be metabolically obese and have hormonal imbalance. I recommend increasing physical activity to seven hours each week—an average of one hour every day. This may seem like a lot, but any type of physical activity counts—shopping, cleaning, gardening, or walking. You don't have to do it all at one time. You can get 10 minutes in the morning, 20 minutes at lunch, and 30 minutes in the evening. Every little bit counts. If you are out of shape and have increased body fat, increasing your level of physical activity will reverse hormonal imbalance and will help you live a healthier and longer life.

Never Feel Hungry

The normal response of a diet is to make leptin and adiponectin levels fall. When these hormone levels go down, your appetite increases and your metabolic rate slows down. If you want to lose weight and keep it off, you have to improve how efficiently your hormones work. By doing so, as you lose weight and as hormone levels go down, less food intake will be needed to keep your appetite under control. The Leptin Boost Diet will help you lose weight while decreasing leptin resistance and increasing adiponectin levels. This will enable you to lose weight without hunger or cravings.

Side Effects of Weight Loss

As with anything in life, weight loss can have its complications, or side effects. Most of the side effects of the Leptin Boost Diet are minor and temporary. I always tell my patients that the No. 1 side effect of weight loss is feeling better—a good thing! And it's true for the vast majority of patients. Some, however, may experience a few temporary side effects. Being aware of possible side effects of weight loss is important because, when armed with that knowledge, you can prevent anxiety, deal with the problems, and move on.

When you lose weight you are losing water. You can't prevent it. This is a normal part of weight loss. People who are very successful at losing weight are at higher risk of getting dehydrated. It is therefore extremely important that you drink plenty of water when you are losing weight. This prevents the dehydration and keeps you feeling good. When you get dehydrated, you feel tired and your weight loss will slow down. The metabolic machinery cannot function properly if you are dehydrated. Other symptoms of dehydration include headache, constipation, dizziness on standing, dry mouth, dry skin, and excessive thirst.

It is also common to have a change in your bowel pattern when you lose weight. This makes sense. Different food going in—different aftermath coming out. The Leptin Boost Diet is very high in fiber because of the number of fruits and vegetables, so it is unusual for someone to become constipated. Still, sometimes bloating, flatulence, and loose stools are a side effect. If you have these symptoms, try different vegetables and fruits, and try eating fewer raw vegetables. You may also want to try one of the over-the-counter enzyme supplements that help you digest vegetables.

If you have high blood pressure or diabetes, it is likely that you will need an adjustment in your medications as you lose weight. This is a major positive side effect, but it means that you should see your doctor regularly. Many medications need dosage adjustments if you change your diet. Typical of these are blood thinners, heart medications, seizure medications, and others. If you take medications of any type, it's wise to discuss your weight-loss plans with your physician.

Another side effect of weight loss is gallstones or a gallbladder attack that is serious enough to require emergency surgery. The risk for this problem is as high as 20 percent and increases according to how much weight you are losing. If you are planning on losing more than 20 pounds, you should be tracked closely by your physician, who can prescribe a medication called Actigall (ursodiol), approved for the prevention of gallstones in a weight-loss program, which can lower your risk of gallstones to about 2 percent.

Details of the Leptin Boost Diet

The Leptin Boost Diet is designed to help you achieve hormonal balance. This diet will improve leptin, adiponectin, insulin, and *all* your hormones to help you lose weight without hunger or cravings. This diet is for anyone—whether you want to lose weight, maintain your weight, or balance your hormones. The Leptin Boost Diet uses *exchanges* to keep track of each food group. Dietitians and nutritionists use exchanges as a way of giving nutritional recommendations for their clients. An exchange is a term used to describe specific portion sizes of different foods to supply comparable calories and nutrition. Exchanges are a great way to keep track of both the amount of food and the type of food you eat.

EXCHANGES FOR THE LEPTIN BOOST DIET		
Type of Food	**Weight Loss** Minimum Exchanges	**Weight Maintenance** Minimum Exchanges
Fruit	5	5
Vegetables	5	5
Dairy	0–3	0–4
Starches	0–4	0–6
Proteins	6–8	6–10
Fats	0–2	0–14

There are no strict numbers for exchanges in the Leptin Boost Diet. Instead, there are *minimums* and *maximums* for each exchange. It is very important to eat all the minimum amounts every day, and not to eat more than the maximum allowed.

You can choose from plenty of food, though. Fruits, vegetables, egg whites, and low-calorie weight-loss shakes can be consumed in unlimited amounts. And they should be. You should always make sure that you eat five servings of vegetables and five servings of fruit every day, but more is definitely better.

It seems strange to think that eating more food will help you lose weight, but that is exactly what I am saying. The key is to intentionally overeat healthy foods so that you feel satisfied and full all the time. You should never feel hungry.

Many people may believe that this sounds like a crazy fad diet. I assure you it's not. The Leptin Boost Diet has helped thousands of people achieve hormonal balance and permanent weight loss. This diet may be difficult in the beginning, because many people are not used to eating this quantity of vegetables and fruits. Eventually, you will adjust to this way of eating and will feel bad if you return to your old eating habits.

In the beginning it will be a challenge to eat all your minimums. If you aren't used to eating five fruits and five vegetables daily, you may want to start off with a transition period, gradually increasing to the full diet over a couple of weeks. I've had many patients lose a significant amount of weight even if they don't follow the diet completely, but they usually don't lose all the weight they want to lose unless they follow the diet more precisely. I strongly encourage you to do your utmost to eat all your exchanges. These foods will eliminate hunger and cravings and will give your body the nutrients it needs for hormonal balance and a healthy metabolism:

- Vegetables (minimum 5 servings per day)
- Fruits (minimum 5 servings per day)
- Egg Whites
- Low-Calorie Diet Shakes

The Leptin Boost Diet has three meals and three snacks a day. It is imperative that you eat six times a day. Smaller frequent meals keep your hormones in balance and prevent undue hunger and cravings.

You must eat protein early in the day—at breakfast and the morning snack. Protein in the morning supplies energy and reduces hunger for the entire day. Your lunch and the mid-afternoon snack should be lighter. The dinner should be balanced with protein and lots of vegetables. The evening snack is imperative to help maintain your metabolism during the night.

1 Protein Exchange = 7 grams of protein (35 calories)

1 Starch Exchange = 15 grams of carbohydrate (60 calories)

1 Fat Exchange = 5 grams of fat (45 calories)

The exact numbers aren't critical. Rather, this breakdown should be used as a rough guide to getting in the right amount and combinations of foods. You should use these recommendations as a way to design your own meal plan. The most important thing is to get in your minimums and to eat all day long.

Eating Frequently Maximizes Leptin Efficiency

Break the Feast–Famine Cycle: Convince Your Body It's Not Starving

"Eat more to lose more." This doesn't inherently make sense. Most people just don't believe it. In my experience treating thousands of overweight patients, one of the biggest mistakes I've seen is that people don't eat frequently enough. It's been engraved in our minds since we were children. "Don't snack." "Snacking makes you gain weight." "Eat three square meals a day." I've even seen a book written about leptin that mistakenly instructs the readers to increase the time between meals in order to lose weight.

The truth is that studies have consistently shown that the *more* meals you have per day, the *less* likely you are to be overweight. In fact, some of my more obese patients, weighing in excess of 400 pounds, have told me they usually only eat once a day. It's the lean, healthy patients who eat all day long.

Infrequent eating is the way sumo wrestlers gain weight. Sumo wrestlers often weigh well over 400 pounds, a handy size to be when you're trying to win a match. But they gain all that weight by skipping breakfast and eating a huge lunch. They know that if they eat breakfast, they won't be able to eat as much rice, vegetables, and meat during the lunchtime feast.

If you want to lose fat and replace it with muscle, you have to go beyond just eating the right foods. You have to give your body a constant source of energy. You need to eat more often. It's a hard concept to grasp—eat more often to weigh less. Eating smaller meals more constantly revs up your body's metabolic machinery and puts you in fat-burning mode. It helps leptin work at its maximum efficiency, convincing your brain that you're not starving.

When you eat three meals a day, your body becomes accustomed to getting nutrients at fairly long intervals. You go several hours between meals. Leptin levels plummet and metabolism slows to conserve energy. By the time the next meal comes around, you feel sluggish but ravenous. It's a mini feast–famine cycle. You eat a substantial meal (the feast), and then wait several hours (the famine) until your next meal. The end result is that leptin stays low, driving up your appetite and cravings.

Eventually, the body goes into starvation mode. It doesn't know when it's going to get the next meal. Leptin production goes into hibernation and so does your metabolism. Your metabolic machinery, which has evolved over hundreds of generations, is still focused on protecting you from starvation. Your body doesn't understand that if you go a few hours between meals the next famine is not right around the corner. Your body makes leptin the same way it has for generations. Leptin's main function is to protect you from starving. Leptin behaves as if you are in a famine, even when you aren't. Our hormones haven't caught up with modern civilization. The result is that the same mechanism that once protected us from starvation is making us fat.

To end this cycle, you have to convince your body that you are not starving. The best way to do this is to give it a constant supply of food. By eating every few hours, your leptin production will increase and so will your metabolism. Your body won't think it's facing the next famine. Your insulin will stop its daily roller coaster ride that follows larger meals. You will have decreased hunger and more energy.

Admittedly, it's not easy to eat small meals all day long. Our society has evolved into one that accommodates breakfast, lunch, and dinner. Our daily lives revolve around the three meals. And unless you have a personal chef to follow you around all day, it takes a great deal of effort and planning. Some people tell me they feel a sense of loss if they don't have that traditional large dinner every night. It's as if the old friend they've grown up with is gone. But along with losing old habits, you *will* lose weight. As you continue to eat small meals frequently throughout the day, your body will begin to change. You won't have excessive hunger or cravings, and your metabolism will be supercharged.

The Importance of Breakfast

Many studies have linked obesity to skipping breakfast. Once you see leptin, it's easy to see why. If you forego breakfast, it's likely that you are going 16 to 18 hours per day without food. During that time, the body stops making leptin, metabolism slows down considerably, and appetite and cravings increase.

Many of my patients have told me that they simply aren't hungry for breakfast. In reply, I tell them that I've found the most common reason for not being hungry for breakfast to be overeating at dinner. Yet another vicious cycle. When people skip breakfast, they get too hungry for lunch and dinner and so they eat too much. By eating frequently, you can break this cycle and be hungry for breakfast.

When you eat breakfast, you supercharge your metabolism. Your leptin will stay up, keeping down appetite and cravings. You should always eat protein with breakfast. That will reduce appetite for the entire day. Many people make the mistake of eating mostly carbohydrates for breakfast. They have cereal and skim milk, juice and toast, oatmeal or a bagel. On the surface, these breakfasts don't seem too bad, but they are very unbalanced. If your breakfast is mostly carbohydrates, it causes problems with insulin spiking and blood sugar crashes. This sends leptin into a downward spiral, making you feel ravenous around midmorning and increasing the carbohydrate cravings toward late afternoon. By adding protein to your breakfast, you are balancing the nutrients and preventing these hormonal swings. Your appetite and cravings will diminish and you'll have greater energy during the day.

Slow Digestion Means Fast Metabolism

The glycemic index is a method of rating carbohydrates based on how fast they are digested and how fast sugar enters the bloodstream. An entire industry has developed based on creating low-glycemic index foods—those with slowly digested carbohydrates. Slow digestion helps the body cope with your meals. When you eat foods that are digested slowly, you're giving your hormones a chance to work at their maximum efficiency.

It's no different than the concept of eating frequently during the day. Both provide a constant source of nutrients to the body. If you eat foods that take several hours to digest, you'll be sitting down at your next meal or snack before the last one has left your system. The idea is to keep the nutrients coming in at a constant rate. This shifts your hormones out of starvation mode, decreases appetite, and speeds the metabolism. The food you eat will be then burned as energy instead of being stored as fat.

If digestion of carbohydrates is speeded up, there's a huge rush of sugar into the blood, causing insulin to spike and leptin to plummet. This causes the sugar to be converted into fat, instead of energy, and results in a rapid lowering of blood sugar, along with feelings of fatigue.

Some fad diets promote certain combinations of foods to speed up digestion. Any diet that combines specific foods for the purposes of enhancing digestion is fundamentally flawed. So beware of diets that base their food combinations on enhancing digestion: all they're doing is overloading your hormonal systems, and that will actually make you gain weight, not lose it.

Increase Volume: Maximize Your Gut Hormones

Feeling "Full" Versus Feeling "Not Hungry"

You can't be successful losing weight and keeping it off unless your appetite is satisfied. Hunger is your brain's way of telling the body it is starving, even if it is not really true. Hunger is very powerful indeed. In a contest between hunger and willpower, hunger will win every time. If you want to lose weight and keep it off, you have to satisfy your appetite. But your goal is more than just to satisfy hunger. You should actually eat until you feel very full, all the time. When you eat until you feel full, you maximize the hunger-quenching effect of your intestinal hormones and can override some of the hunger problems caused by leptin resistance, low adiponectin, and other hormonal problems. You can harness the power of your gut hormones to see an immediate effect on appetite and cravings that will eventually have long-term benefits for your weight. You can take advantage of gut hormones to supersede the appetite stimulation caused by leptin resistance and low adiponectin levels.

One study examined women eating a pasta meal. On one day they were given a meal of pasta primavera that had a lot of pasta and high-fat sauce with very few vegetables. On a different day, the same women were given a meal of pasta primavera that had less pasta, less low-fat sauce, and lots of vegetables. The women ate the same amount of food at both meals—about two pounds. The women reported feeling equally full and satisfied after both meals. Even so, the women ate about 500 calories less with the high-vegetable pasta, compared to the low-vegetable pasta. Many other studies have had similar results. Your feelings of fullness come more from the volume and amount of the food you eat, rather than the ingredients of the meal.

When your belly is full, intestinal hormones respond. Ghrelin levels drop and there's a surge of glucagon-like peptide-1, cholecystokinin, and peptide YY levels. This is your digestive system's way of communicating with your brain. For the most part, these hormones respond to how distended your stomach and intestines are. It's not so much *what* you eat as how *much* you eat.

Digestive hormones respond at a moment's notice. Unlike leptin, adiponectin, and the other fat hormones, the digestive hormones are more concerned with the day-to-day food you put in your body. Digestive hormones are short-term regulators of appetite and satiety. So, when you eat to change these hormones, the effect will be short-lived. To maximize the effect of these hormones, you have to make permanent changes in your diet.

There's no reason to feel hungry when you are trying to lose weight. If you do, there's a good chance that you will not be successful. You can't fight against your hormones; you have to work with them. To balance your intestinal hormones and your appetite, you have to eat high volumes of low-calorie foods. This will keep ghrelin levels low and levels of glucagon-like peptide-1, cholecystokinin, and peptide YY high.

You can take advantage of your gut hormones to maximize weight loss. It's important to not be hungry when you are losing weight, but there's a difference between simply not feeling hungry and feeling full. Feeling full is really much better. At first, most people think this is an absurd notion. Eat more to lose weight? Overeat to lose weight? Yes.

When you intentionally overeat healthy foods, you will maximize the power of your gut hormones. You can take advantage of these hormones to overpower the effects that other hormones have on your appetite. If you have leptin resistance, for example, the natural response is to feel hungry all the time. The brain doesn't see leptin so it is fooled into thinking the body is starving. Hunger is chronically elevated. Gut hormones can override the increased appetite caused by leptin resistance to help you feel full and satisfied. Gut hormones tell the body you're not starving, despite the brain's inability to see leptin. By taking advantage of your gut hormones, you will lose weight and leptin resistance will improve. Your hunger and cravings will improve as well. But it's always hard work. Due to the short-term nature of gut hormones, you have to deal with them every day and with every meal.

When you aren't hungry, you can still eat. People eat out of stress, boredom, or depression, not always out of hunger—but they still eat. When you eat a delicious meal and feel totally satisfied, you may still eat the dessert that's placed in front of you. If you're completely full, it's a different story. When you feel full, your gut hormones are telling your brain "no more." It's difficult to eat anything at all. You will not have hunger or cravings and you'll regain control of your appetite. You can plan your meals to be healthy meals that will allow you to feel totally satisfied. You can regain control over the food you put in your body. And it's all because you have learned to harness the power of the hormones made by your gut.

It takes hard work to keep yourself feeling full. You have to fight against your body's signals. You have to eat when you're not hungry. The Leptin Boost Diet was developed with this principle in mind. You should start eating early in the day. You should consume at least the minimum amount of food every day, and if you're hungry you need to eat more. But don't let yourself get hungry. Just keep eating. The more you eat, the more weight you'll lose.

Caloric Density of Food

The caloric density of food is a concept used to describe the number of calories in a particular food, compared to the food's weight or volume. When a particular food is described as "high-calorie" or "low-calorie," the reference is really to its caloric density. When it comes to losing weight, the foods with the lowest caloric density are the best way to go. These are the foods that are high in volume and low in calories.

Low-caloric-density foods include:
- vegetables
- fruits
- whole-grain foods
- low-fat or fat-free dairy products
- high-fiber foods
- weight-loss shakes
- low-fat proteins
- egg whites & egg substitutes

These are the foods that will help you feel full and satisfied without causing you to gain weight. These foods maximize your gut hormones, in turn quenching appetite and eliminating your body's cravings.

Carbohydrates

Although some fad diets emphasize low- or no-carbohydrate intake, carbohydrates are an important part of your diet and are critical for hormonal balance. Carbohydrates come in two types: simple and complex. Simple carbohydrates are sugars; complex carbohydrates are starches. Regardless of what kind they are, carbohydrates—in the form of sugar, wheat, rice, grains, fruit, and vegetables—are the main components of our diet. We all need carbohydrates in our diet. But to achieve hormonal balance, the majority of the carbohydrates that you eat should be the healthy variety. In fact, most of the carbohydrates in your diet should come from fruits and vegetables.

Vegetables and Fruits

When it comes to leptin and hormonal balance, vegetables and fruits are the best carbohydrates that you can eat. If there's such a thing as a "miracle food" for weight loss, vegetables and fruits are just that. *The Leptin Boost Diet* allows you to have unlimited amounts of most fruits and vegetables. Why? They're extremely low in calories. It is next to impossible to gain weight by eating unlimited quantities of fruits and vegetables. In fact the opposite is true: the more vegetables and fruits you eat, the more weight you're likely to lose. Vegetables and fruits are high in fiber and antioxidants. Research has documented the effect of vegetables and fruits on the reduction of cancer, cardiovascular disease, diabetes, and other medical problems.

I recommend that you eat at least 5 servings of fruits and 5 servings of vegetables every day. But more is better! If you're hungry, eat more vegetables and fruits. It's better if you have only fresh vegeta-

---

VEGETABLE EXCHANGES

A serving of vegetables is 1 cup of fresh vegetables or ½ cup cooked. You should have a minimum of 5 servings of vegetables every day.

Artichoke	Lettuce
Asparagus	Mushrooms
Beans	Okra
Beets	Onions
Broccoli	Pea pods
Brussels sprouts	Peppers
Cabbage	Pumpkin
Cauliflower	Radishes
Celery	Spinach
Cucumber	Sprouts
Eggplant	Squash
Greens	Tomato
Heart of palm	Turnips
Leeks	Zucchini

FRUIT EXCHANGES

You should have a minimum of 5 servings of fruit every day.

Fruit	Quantity	Fruit	Quantity
Apple	1 small	Limes	2
Apricots	4 whole	Mango	½
Banana	1 small	Nectarine	1
Blackberries	¾ cup	Orange	1 small
Blueberries	¾ cup	Peach	1 medium
Cantaloupe	¼ of 6" melon	Pear (1 cup, cubed)	1 small
Cherries chopped	12	Pineapple, fresh	1/2 cup
Grapefruit	½	Plums	2
Grapes	17	Raspberries	1 cup
Honeydew	⅛ of 7" melon	Strawberries (1 cup, cubed)	1¼ cup
Kiwi	1	Tangerine	2
Lemons	2	Watermelon	4" x ½" or 1¼ cups cubed

bles and fruits (although frozen or canned in unsweetened juice is also acceptable). Dried fruits, sweetened canned fruits, and fruit juices are high in calories and are like processed carbohydrates and therefore are not as healthy. Many people who are not used to eating vegetables and fruits have trouble eating this much on a daily basis. I encourage you to keep trying. Eventually you will get used to eating 10 servings of vegetables and fruits each day. When you fill your stomach with these healthy foods, you will feel full and satisfied all day long.

A serving of fruit depends on the fruit. Although I recommend that you eat as much fruit as possible, some people with diabetes or prediabetes may need to limit the amount they eat. Consuming a minimum of 5 servings per day doesn't seem to be a problem for most people, but some of my patients with diabetes have noticed blood sugar elevations when they eat more fruit, especially bananas, grapes, mangos, pineapple, or watermelon. I recommend that you don't eat more than 5 servings total for such fruits each day. Overall, though, all fruit is extremely healthful and most people can eat as much as they want.

On the Leptin Boost Diet, canned fruit, dried fruit, and fruit juices are not a substitute for fresh or frozen fruit. Processed fruits are very high in sugar and should only be consumed in limited amounts. The following lists portion sizes for processed fruits. You should count these foods as carbohydrates and *not* fruit, when following the Leptin Boost Diet.

PROCESSED FRUIT EXCHANGES

Processed fruits should only be eaten in small amounts. You should count processed fruits as a carbohydrate exchange and not a fruit exchange.

Juices	Quantity	Dried Fruits	Quantity
Apple	½ cup	Apricots	8 halves
Grape	⅓ cup	Apples	4 rings
Grapefruit	½ cup	Dates	3 small
Lemon	½ cup	Figs	3 small
Orange	½ cup	Mango slices	4 strips
Prune	⅓ cup	Peaches	2 halves
		Pears	3 halves
Other		Prunes	4 medium
Applesauce	½ cup	Raisins	2 Tbsp
Fruit cocktail (unsweetened)	¾ cup		
Pineapple (crushed, in own juice)	½ cup		
Pineapple rings	2		
Jam or jelly, low-sugar	2 tsp 2 tsp		
Syrup, sugar-free	2 Tbsp		

Healthy Carbohydrates

The glycemic index is a valuable tool in learning to avoid spikes in blood sugar levels that will help balance both leptin and insulin. The glycemic index was developed in 1981 by David Jenkins and Thomas Wolever. These doctors found that not all carbohydrate foods are digested at equal rates, meaning that sugar is released into the bloodstream at varying rates. Foods with a higher glycemic index pump sugar into the bloodstream quickly, while foods with a lower glycemic index are digested slowly and release sugar gradually.

Unhealthy carbohydrates contain finely milled wheat. By milling out wheat bran and wheat germ, these products have been stripped of vital minerals, vitamins, fiber, and proteins. The white flour in these products is rapidly digested and causes blood sugar spikes. Complex carbohydrates are healthier and are digested more slowly. These include whole and unprocessed grains, foods high in fiber, vegetables, and fruits.

The glycemic index is a number determined by measuring blood sugar levels in volunteer subjects who eat 50 grams of a particular carbohydrate food. The amount of food varies, as long as it contains 50 grams of carbohydrate. The lower the score, the healthier the carbohydrate. Foods with a glycemic index score of 70 or above are considered to be high, scores between 56 and 69 are moderate, and scores of 55 or less are considered low.

GLYCEMIC INDEX AND GLYCEMIC LOAD		
	Glycemic index	Glycemic load
High	above 70	above 20
Moderate	56–69	11–19
Low	below 55	below 10

Although important, the glycemic index doesn't tell the whole story about the impact of glucose in the bloodstream. The *glycemic load* provides a more accurate picture. The glycemic load takes into account other factors, namely the average portion size of the food. Foods with higher fiber tend to have the lowest glycemic load scores. When fiber is ingested, it makes you feel full—it makes the stomach swell. This fiber slows gastric emptying, keeping the food in the stomach longer. As a result, leptin works more efficiently and adiponectin levels rise. A glycemic load of 20 or more is considered high, between 11 and 19 is moderate, and 10 or below is considered low.

Carbohydrates are often blamed for failed weight-loss attempts. That's because most people eat too many carbohydrates, especially the unhealthy ones. It's OK to eat carbohydrates, but the main source should be fruits and vegetables. Recommended carbohydrates are:

- Fruits
- High-Fiber Foods
- Low-Fat Dairy Products
- Low Glycemic Index and Glycemic Load Foods
- Soy Products
- Vegetables
- Whole-Grain Products

The carbohydrates listed below should be eaten only in limited amounts.

CARBOHYDRATE EXCHANGES

Starch	Quantity	Starch	Quantity
Bread: white, wheat French, rye, pumpernickel	1 slice	Matzo	1 square, 5x5"
Bagel	½	Fat-free muffin	1 small
Biscuit or roll (low-fat)	1 small	Melba toast	4
Breadcrumbs	¼ cup	Pasta	½ cup
Breadsticks	1½ cup	Peas	½
Bun, hamburger or frankfurter	½	Pita bread	1 small
Cooked cereal	½ cup	Popcorn (air popped)	3 cups
Puffed cereal	1½ cup	White potato	1 small or ½ cup mashed
Bran cereal	½ cup		
Unsweetened, ready-to-eat cereal	¾ cup	Sweet potato	½ cup
		Pretzels	½ cup
Corn	½ cup or 1 small ear	Rice	½ cup
		Rice cakes	2
Graham crackers	3 x 2½" squares	Tortilla small	1
Oyster crackers	½ cup		
Saltine crackers	6		
Soda crackers	6		
Macaroni noodles (cooked)	½ cup		
English muffin	½		

GLYCEMIC INDEX AND GLYCEMIC LOAD OF SELECTED FOODS

From the International Table of Glycemic Index and from *Overcoming Metabolic Syndrome* (Addicus Books)

	Glycemic Index	Glycemic Load
Breads		
Bagel, white, frozen	72	25
Baguette, white, frozen	95	15
Bread stuffing	74	16
Barley kernel bread, 50% barley flour	46	9
Barley flour bread, 100% barley flour	67	9
Coarse whole wheat bread	52	10
Hamburger bun	61	9
Melba toast	70	16
Gluten-free white bread (gluten-free wheat starch)	76	11
Oat bran bread	47	9
Rye kernel (pumpernickel) bread	50	6
Whole meal rye bread	58	8
White wheat flour bread	70	10
Pita bread	57	10
Crackers		
Breton wheat crackers	64	10
Puffed rice cakes	78	17
Rye crackers	64	11
Stoned wheat crackers	67	12
Soda crackers	74	12
Breakfast Cereals		
All-Bran	42	9
Bran Buds	58	7
Bran Flakes	74	13
Cheerios	74	15
Corn Flakes	81	21
Cream of Wheat	66	17
Golden Grahams	71	18

	Glycemic Index	Glycemic Load
Grapenuts	71	15
Mini Wheats, whole wheat	58	12
Muesli	49	10
Nutrigrain	66	10
Oat bran	67	9
Quick Oats	66	17
Puffed wheat	67	13
Raisin Bran	61	12
Rice Krispies	82	21
Shredded Wheat	75	15
Total	76	13
Wheat biscuits (plain flaked wheat)	70	13
Cereal Grains		
Pearl barley	25	7
Buckwheat	54	16
Cornmeal	69	9
Sweet corn	53	17
Couscous	65	23
Millet	71	25
Rice, white	64	23
Rice, brown	55	18
Instant, puffed rice	69	29
Pastas		
Fettuccine	40	18
Linguine	46	22
Mung bean noodles	33	15
Macaroni	47	23
Spaghetti, white, boiled	42	20
Vermicelli, white, boiled	35	16
Fruits		
Apples, raw	38	6
Apricots, raw	57	5
Apricots, canned in light syrup	64	12
Apricots, dried	30	16
Banana, raw	51	13
Cantaloupe	65	4
Cherries, raw	22	3

	Glycemic Index	Glycemic Load
Cranberry juice	68	16
Dates, dried	103	42
Figs, dried	61	16
Grapes, raw	59	11
Kiwi fruit, raw	53	6
Lychee, canned in syrup and drained	79	16
Mango, raw	51	8
Oranges, raw	42	5
Papaya, raw	59	7
Peaches	42	5
Pears	38	4
Pineapple	59	7
Plums	39	5
Prunes, pitted	29	10
Raisins	64	28
Strawberries	40	1
Tomato juice	38	4
Watermelon, raw	72	4
Vegetables		
Green peas	54	4
Pumpkin	75	3
Carrots	47	3
Sweet corn	62	11
Parsnips	97	12
Boiled potato	50	14
French fries	75	22
Mashed potato	91	18
Sweet potato	61	17
Tapioca	70	12
Taro	55	4
Yam	37	13
Legumes		
Baked beans	48	7
Beans, dried, boiled	29	9
Black-eyed peas	42	13
Butter beans	31	6

	Glycemic Index	Glycemic Load
Chickpeas (Garbanzo beans, Bengal gram), boiled	28	8
Navy beans	38	12
Kidney beans	28	7
Lentils	29	5
Lima beans	32	10
Mung beans	31	5
Peas, dried, boiled	22	2
Pinto beans	39	10
Soybeans	18	1
Split peas	32	6
Beverages		
Coca-Cola	58	15
Apple juice	40	12
Carrot juice	43	11
Cranberry juice cocktail	56	16
Grapefruit juice, unsweetened	48	11
Orange juice	50	13
Pineapple juice, unsweetened	46	16
Tomato juice	38	4
Gatorade	8	12
Hot chocolate mix	51	11
Water	0	0
Dairy Products		
Custard	38	6
Ice cream, regular	61	8
Ice cream, reduced or low-fat	39	5
Ice cream, premium	38	3
Milk, full-fat	27	3
Milk, skim	32	4
Chocolate milk	34	9
Pudding	44	7
Yogurt	36	3
Yogurt, low-fat with aspartame	14	2
Nuts		
Cashews	22	3
Peanuts	14	1

Dairy Products

An important part of the Leptin Boost Diet are dairy products. Besides protein and carbohydrates, dairy products contain a lot of calcium and vitamin D. Only one third of Americans get enough calcium. Calcium is best known for keeping bones healthy and strong, but recent research has also shown that calcium can help you lose weight. Calcium makes cells less likely to store fat and more likely to burn fat, when calories are reduced. Too little calcium in the diet slows metabolism, decreases fat burning, and increases fat storage. A recent review of several scientific studies, published in the *Journal of the American College of Nutrition,* concluded that people who consume less calcium tend to be more overweight and gain more weight later in life. For every 300 milligrams consumed in a day (about an eight-ounce glass of skim milk), adults tend to weigh about six pounds less.

Researchers recommend that for ideal metabolism and weight loss people should consume about 1,000–1,500 milligrams of calcium daily. (Menopausal women and others with bone problems should consume at least 1,500 milligrams of calcium daily.) The best source for calcium is dairy products. Many dieters give up milk because they think it is fattening, when the opposite may be true. Dairy products often contain fat as well as calcium, so it's important to choose low-fat or fat-free varieties. Calcium is also available in fortified foods such as juices and cereals as well as in tablet form as supplements.

Many varieties of calcium tablets are on the market, but not all contain the same amount of calcium, so it's important to read the label. If you have an allergy to milk or are lactose intolerant, you can eliminate this group from the diet and substitute low-fat proteins or soy milk. Soy milk is an alternative to skim milk, and comes in many different types. The nutritional content varies among the varieties, so it's a good idea, as always, to read the labels.

DAIRY EXCHANGES

Product	Quantity
Skim milk	1 cup
Skim milk (powdered)	⅓ cup
Yogurt (low-fat or fat-free)	1 cup
Plain/light sweetened or fat-free cottage cheese	½ cup
Soy milk (low-fat)	1 cup

By eliminating or restricting milk in the diet, you risk inadequate calcium intake. Most soy milks are fortified with calcium, though may not contain enough. If you have any concerns, you should take a daily calcium supplement.

MAKE A FRUIT SMOOTHIE!

- ½ cup fat-free yogurt or 1 scoop protein powder or weight-loss shake mix
- ⅔ cup fruit (fresh or frozen) (banana, mango, blueberries, blackberries, raspberries, strawberries, peaches, etc.)
- 6 oz cold water
- 3–4 ice cubes

Put water and fruit in blender and turn on low.

Pour in shake mix, protein powder, or yogurt and continue blending on low.

Add ice cubes slowly as it blends. Adding more ice will create a lighter and fluffier smoothie.

When all ingredients are added, secure the lid and blend on low for 1–2 minutes, then on high for 30 seconds.

Smoothies are a great way to get in lots of dairy products as well as fruit. You can experiment with different ingredients. Smoothies will help you feel full and satisfied. They can be used in place of a meal, or in between meals. Studies have shown that people who take snacks like smoothies between meals will lose more weight than those who do not snack. I recommend having one or two smoothies a day. My personal favorite is a blueberry and pineapple smoothie made with fat-free vanilla yogurt.

Protein

You should eat about 0.4 grams of protein each day for every pound
you weigh. So, a 170-pound person should consume about 65–70
grams of protein each day. The Leptin Boost Diet allows for limited
amounts of most proteins but unlimited quantities of egg whites,
egg substitutes, and low-calorie protein shakes. In theory, while this
could lead to eating too much protein, in practice most people find
it difficult to eat too much of these healthy proteins. If you have kid-

PROTEIN EXCHANGES	
Meat/Meat Substitutes	**Quantity (1 oz unless indicated)**
Beef	Lean, trimmed of fat
	Choose round or loin cuts
Pork	Fresh ham, Canadian bacon,
	tenderloin, center loin chop
Poultry	White meat, no skin
Fish	Cod, flounder, grouper, haddock,
	halibut, trout, tuna, salmon,
	snapper, canned tuna or salmon
	in water (¼ cup)
Shellfish	Clams, crab, lobster, scallops,
	shrimp, imitation shellfish
Game	Buffalo, ostrich, venison, deer, elk
Cheese	Less than 3 grams per slice
(non-fat or low-fat)	
Cottage cheese	½ cup
(low-fat or fat-free)	
Egg whites	Unlimited (2 are equivalent to 1
	very lean protein exchange)
Egg substitute	Unlimited (½ cup is equivalent
(fat-free)	to 1 very lean protein exchange)
Whole egg	(1 protein and 1 fat)
Lunch meat (fat-free)	1 oz
Soy:	
Tofu	3 oz
Soy burger	(counts as 2 protein and ½ starch)
Cooked beans	½ cup (1 protein and 1 starch)

ney problems, you should consume much less protein. If you have any doubts, see your doctor.

I recommend that you eat very lean cuts of meat or eat other low-fat sources of protein, such as beans or imitation meat products. A very lean exchange should have zero to one gram of fat. I recommend grilling, baking, or broiling meat to remove all possible fat.

On the Leptin Boost Diet, egg whites, egg substitutes, and low-calorie protein shakes are unlimited. To achieve hormonal balance, your body has to get enough protein. Your body will crave protein and if you don't get enough of it you'll feel hungry all the time. When you consume enough protein, gut hormones work to help you feel full and satisfied. Eating sufficient protein also helps preserve muscle and maintains a healthy metabolism. Egg whites, egg substitutes, and low-calorie protein shakes are a great way to make sure your body is getting enough protein and help you to maintain hormonal balance.

Protein and Gut Hormones

Protein is vitally important for the Leptin Boost Diet because it directs your gut hormones to shut down your appetite. Protein decreases production of the appetite-stimulating hormone ghrelin, and it increases levels of appetite-lowering hormones such as glucagon-like peptide-1, cholecystokinin, and peptide YY. When the intestinal tract sees protein, gut hormones go into action. This is why so many experts recommend increasing protein to lose weight. Foods like fruits, vegetables, and other high-fiber foods swell in the stomach and can stimulate gut hormones in a similar way to protein, but their effect doesn't last nearly as long. I always recommend that you eat protein in the morning. When you do so then, your gut hormones go into overdrive, keeping hunger at a minimum all day long.

Protein in the Morning

You must eat protein at breakfast. This is a change for most people who are not accustomed to eating protein in the morning. Most people eat pure (or mostly) carbohydrate breakfasts such as toast and juice, cold cereal or oatmeal, waffles or pancakes. A high-carb load in the morning causes blood sugar spiking and results in hunger and carbohydrate cravings. In fact, these symptoms are so common that many people skip breakfast to avoid the mid-morning crash. The problem is that skipping breakfast causes problems with leptin and insulin. Eating protein for breakfast will help control appetite and cravings during the whole day.

RECOMMENDED PROTEINS	
Beans	Elk
Beef, lean, grass-fed	Fish
Buffalo	Ostrich
Chicken breast	Oysters
Clams	Scallops
Cottage cheese, fat-free	Shrimp
Deer	Soy products
Egg whites	Turkey, lean

Fat

An important part of our diet is fat. The right types of fats are important for hormonal balance. A *balanced* diet means a healthy blend of carbohydrates, protein, and fat. Diets that are very low or very high in fat, or high in trans or saturated fat, cause leptin and adiponectin problems. But diets that have 25 to 35 percent fat, which is mostly healthy fat, enable your fat cell hormones to be balanced so that they will function at their maximum capacity.

I recommend that your diet have about 25 to 35 percent fat. Fat helps you feel full and will balance blood sugar levels by slowing down the rate at which the entire meal hits the bloodstream, thus slowing digestion. Plus, fat makes the digestive tract produce hormones—like cholecystokinin, glucagon-like peptide 1, peptide YY, and others—that tell your brain that it's full. Fat shuts down production of the hunger hormone, ghrelin. Fat makes you feel full.

All fats have the same number of calories—9 calories per gram. This is twice as many calories as protein or carbohydrates. Even "healthy fat" is still fat.

FAT EXCHANGES	
Monounsaturated Fat	**Quantity**
Oil (canola, olive, peanut)	1/8 tsp
Olives: ripe (black)	8 large green, stuffed 10 large
Nuts	
almonds, cashews	6
mixed	6
pecans	4 halves
Peanut butter	2 tsp
Sesame seeds	1 Tbsp
Polyunsaturated Fat	**Quantity**
Margarine: stick, tub, or squeeze	1 tsp
Lower-fat (30 to 50% vegetable oil)	1 Tbsp
Mayonnaise (reduced-fat)	2 Tbsp
Nuts, walnuts	4 halves
Oil (corn, safflower, soybean)	1 tsp
Salad dressing (reduced-fat)	2 Tbsp
Miracle Whip salad dressing (reduced fat)	1 Tbsp
Seeds: pumpkin, sunflower	1 Tbsp

Healthy Fat

We consider healthy fats to be an important part of hormonal balance. Studies have shown that eating healthy fats will increase the size of the mitochondria in your cells. These tiny "powerhouses" are the cellular machinery responsible for energy production and metabolism. This helps increase metabolism and increase energy levels.

Healthy fats are also known as *unsaturated fats*. Fish, avocados, olives, seeds, and nuts are good sources of unsaturated fat. Chicken breast meat has some unsaturated fat, but chicken skin and thigh meat has more saturated fat. Grass-fed beef and meat from other animals, as well as buffalo, elk, and deer, has a more unsaturated fat than does grain-fed beef. Olive oil, peanut oil, sunflower oil, and canola oil are the best oils to use, but all oils should be used with moderation. All fats are high in calories, and calories always matter.

Two fats, linoleic acid and lenolenic acid, are absolutely vital to hormonal balance. They are known as essential fatty acids (EFAs). Without EFAs, you will develop symptoms of essential fatty acid deficiency, like weakness, arthritis, numbness and tingling, dry flaking skin, hair loss, and incoordination.

Omega-3 fatty acids are important for lowering both leptin resistance and insulin resistance. Fish that live in cold water, such as salmon, cod, and halibut, are extremely high in omega-3 fatty acids. Flax, soybeans, sunflower seeds, sesame seeds, peanuts, and walnuts are also good sources of omega-3 fatty acids. Prescription and over-the-counter formulations of omega-3 fatty acids are available as well.

SOURCES OF HEALTHY FAT	
Avocados	Fish
Beef, lean, grass-fed	Nuts
Buffalo	Olives and olive oil
Canola oil	Ostrich
Chicken breast	Seeds
Deer	Peanut oil
Elk	Sunflower oil

Unhealthy fats are *saturated fats* and *trans fats*. These fats are linked to cardiovascular disease, diabetes, cancer, and other problems. These fats come from animal products, tropical oils (like palm oil or coconut oil), or processed oils (like margarine or partially hydrogenated vegetable oil).

Free Foods

You must never be hungry on the Leptin Boost Diet. If you are hungry, your body is telling you that you need to eat more food. The following table lists the foods that you can eat in unlimited amounts. These foods will not make you gain weight. Of course, I'm not sug-

FREE FOODS	
Bouillon (be careful of high sodium content)	Gelatin dessert, sugar-free
	Herbs, fresh or dried
Club soda or mineral water	Mustard
Coffee	Pepper rings, hot
Diet shakes (low-calorie)	Pickles
Diet soft drinks (best to limit to 1 or 2 per day)	Protein shakes, low-calorie
	Pudding, fat-free, sugar-free
Egg whites	Salsa
Egg substitutes	Soy sauce
Fat-free cottage cheese	Spices
Fat-free sour cream	Sugar substitutes
Fat-free, sugar-free yogurt	Tea
Flavoring extracts	Vegetables
Fruit	Vinegar
Garlic	Worcestershire sauce

gesting that you go out and down a whole bottle of Worcestershire sauce. You should always use good common sense, as well.

Foods to Avoid

You should avoid unhealthy fats (saturated fats and trans fats) as much as possible. These fats come from animal products, tropical oils (like palm oil or coconut oil), or processed oils (like margarine

FOODS TO AVOID AS MUCH AS POSSIBLE	
Butter	High-fructose corn syrup
Candy	High-sugar foods and beverages
Chips	Junk food
Dried fruits/fruit roll-ups	Margarine
Fast food	Processed white foods (bread, cake,
Fatty meat	cookies, crackers, mashed potatoes,
Fried foods	french fries, rice, pasta)
Fruit juices	Regular soda
Ground beef	Saturated fat
High-calorie foods	Trans fat
High-fat foods	Tropical oils (coconut, palm)

or partially hydrogenated vegetable oil). You should also stay away from products that contain high-fructose corn syrup. This includes sodas and most sweetened products. In general, you should limit consumption of processed foods that contain white flour.

Alcohol and Leptin

Studies have shown that light intake of alcohol has no significant effect on leptin levels in young men and women. Consuming one or two alcoholic drinks per day was found, however, to increase leptin levels in menopausal women by about 25 percent. More than one hundred published studies indicate that small amounts of alcohol are healthy. And, in fact, people who don't drink have more health problems than those who drink a small portion of alcohol every day. Studies consistently show that drinking one or two alcoholic beverages daily can improve longevity and reduce the risk of cancer, heart disease, and a host of other ailments. If you drink more, though, your risk of health problems will increase.

Alcohol contains a lot of calories—seven calories per gram—which is almost as much as fat. If you are trying to lose weight, it is best to avoid alcohol altogether. Even one or two drinks per week

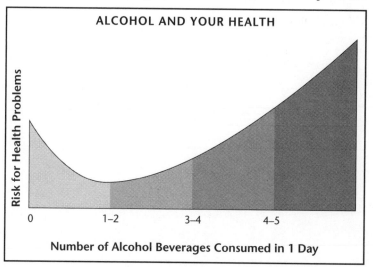

ALCOHOL AND YOUR HEALTH

Risk for Health Problems

0   1–2   3–4   4–5

Number of Alcohol Beverages Consumed in 1 Day

can slow down weight loss considerably. Some people, in fact, will lose weight when they stop drinking, even if they don't change their diet otherwise. Once you reach your weight-loss goal, it is healthy to have one, or on occasion two, alcoholic beverages on a nightly basis. You should not overdo it, though, and you can't save all your drinks up and binge drink on the weekends.

Sample Meal Plan

This meal plan is designed to be a guide for your own customized version of the Leptin Boost Diet. Exact numbers aren't always critical, and you should add as many extra fruits and vegetables as possible. You should always eat a minimum of 5 to 10 servings of vegetables and fruits every day. The quantities of protein will vary according to your weight (see section on protein), and the amounts in this sample meal plan are a rough estimate for the average person. It is important to eat all six meals every day—breakfast, morning snack, lunch, afternoon snack, dinner, and evening snack. Your breakfast should always contain protein.

Variety is the key. The more variety you have, the less it will seem like a diet and the more it will seem a delicious, healthy way of eating. I've suggested a few recipes, which are noted with an asterisk.

DAY 1

BREAKFAST

1 slice whole-grain, high-fiber toast
1 tsp fat-free cream cheese and/or 1 tsp low-sugar marmalade
3 extra-large egg whites, scrambled
2 oz low-fat turkey bacon or low-fat turkey sausage
1 kiwi

MID-MORNING SNACK

1¼ cups watermelon with fat-free feta cheese

LUNCH

Big salad with:
    Salad greens
    3 oz boiled, peeled shrimp or cooked chicken
    3 hard-boiled egg whites (sliced or chopped)
    Cut-up raw vegetables
    Sliced tomato
    1 oz low-fat shredded mozzarella
    Low-fat, reduced-calorie salad dressing
1 large orange or 2 tangerines

MID-AFTERNOON SNACK

1 cup skim milk
3 whole wheat, no-fat/low-fat crisp breads (brands include
    Kavli or Wasa)
1 banana

DINNER

Green salad with low-fat, reduced-calorie dressing
4 oz grilled or broiled fish or chicken
Braised Kale and Yams (page 166)
1 cup steamed vegetables

BEDTIME SNACK

Blueberry pineapple smoothie

DAY 2

BREAKFAST

Egg white omelet with tomatoes, crumbled low-fat turkey
    bacon pieces, and onions

1 whole grapefruit

1 cup skim milk

MID-MORNING SNACK

2 oz fat-free smoked turkey or low-fat turkey ham

¼ cantaloupe or honeydew melon

LUNCH

3 cups Cream of Vegetable Soup (page 167)

1 cup red grapes

MID-AFTERNOON SNACK

Strawberry banana smoothie

DINNER

Salad with low-fat, reduced-calorie dressing

4 oz grilled or broiled beef or turkey tenderloin

3 small red potatoes

1 Tbsp fat-free sour cream (optional)

1 cup steamed vegetables

BEDTIME SNACK

1 cup strawberries, sliced

2 Tbsp fat-free whipped topping (optional)

DAY 3

BREAKFAST

1½ cups breakfast cereal with protein

1 cup skim milk

1 cup berries of choice—strawberries, blueberries, raspberries, blackberries

MID-MORNING SNACK

1 fat-free yogurt with ¼ cup protein cereal as topping

LUNCH

Peasant Salad (page 168)

1 pear or 2 halves sugar-free canned pears (try Del Monte Carb Clever)

MID-AFTERNOON SNACK

Cut-up carrots or baby carrot sticks

Homemade Hummus (page 169)

DINNER

Cut-up ½ avocado and tomato (seasoned with black pepper and lime juice)

4 oz grilled salmon, tuna, or halibut

Roasted Potatoes with Carrots and Onions (page 170)

1 cup steamed vegetables

BEDTIME SNACK

Peach, mango, or pineapple smoothie

DAY 4

BREAKFAST

Scrambled egg white wrap with:

   1 small low-fat tortilla wrap

   4 egg whites scrambled with mushrooms, green peppers, and onion

   1 oz low-fat shredded cheese of choice

   ⅛ cup salsa

   1 Tbsp fat-free sour cream

½ cup sugar-free fruit cocktail (try Del Monte Carb Clever)

MID-MORNING SNACK

Blackberry and raspberry smoothie

LUNCH

1 low-calorie frozen entrée

1 package frozen vegetables

1 large Granny Smith apple

MID-AFTERNOON SNACK

Veggie dip with:

   ½ cup fat-free sour cream

   ½ package fat-free ranch salad dressing mix

   Cut-up carrots, celery, broccoli, peppers, or cucumbers

DINNER

Salad with low-fat, reduced-calorie dressing

4 oz broiled scallops, shrimp, lobster tails, or imitation crab

1 cup steamed squash (spaghetti, summer, zucchini, butternut, acorn, pumpkin, calabaza)

1 cup steamed vegetables

BEDTIME SNACK

Mango Mint Smoothie (page 171)

DAY 5

BREAKFAST

Scrambled egg white sandwich with:

    2 slices whole-grain, high-fiber toast

    4 egg whites, scrambled

    1 oz low-fat cheese

    Lettuce

    Sliced tomato

1 cup cantaloupe or melon

MID-MORNING SNACK

1 fat-free yogurt

1 small banana

LUNCH

Chopped Salad (page 172)

MID-AFTERNOON SNACK

3 oz broiled shrimp with sliced tomato

DINNER

Salad with low-fat, reduced-calorie dressing

4 oz ground turkey, chicken, or veggie burger

¾ cup Black Bean and Corn Salsa (page 173)

½ cup brown rice

1 cup steamed vegetables

BEDTIME SNACK

Lime Pistachio Coconut Smoothie (page 174)

DAY 6

BREAKFAST
1½ cups breakfast cereal with protein
1 cup skim milk
1 cup berries of choice—strawberries, blueberries, raspberries, blackberries
1 oz low-fat cheese

MID-MORNING SNACK
½ cup fat-free cottage cheese
1 cup cut-up fresh fruit

LUNCH
1 reduced-calorie frozen entrée
1 package frozen vegetables

MID-AFTERNOON SNACK
Mini relish tray with:
    Pickles
    hot pepper rings
    carrots
    celery
    cucumbers
    and 2 or 3 olives

DINNER
Salad with low-fat, reduced-calorie dressing
Teriyaki Chicken Kebabs (page 175)
Lemon-Garlic Squash (page 176)
1 cup steamed vegetables

BEDTIME SNACK
1 medium peach
1 cup fat-free yogurt

DAY 7

BREAKFAST

2 slices French toast made with egg whites and whole-grain, high-fiber bread

1 cup skim milk

½ cup fruit of choice

MID-MORNING SNACK

2 sticks celery filled with fat-free cream cheese dotted with ½ oz chopped nuts

LUNCH

Egg salad pita with:

   ½ cup Egg Salad (page 177)

   Sliced tomato

   Sprouts

1 nectarine

MID-AFTERNOON SNACK

1 fat-free yogurt with ¼ cup granola as topping

DINNER

Salad with low-fat, reduced-calorie dressing

1 large Turkey and Rice Stuffed Peppers (page 178)

2 cups steamed vegetables

BEDTIME SNACK

Banana smoothie

Recipes

Braised Kale and Yams
makes 6 servings

1½ lbs kale, coarsely chopped

1 lb yams, ¼-inch dice

8 oz water

½ tsp salt

1 tsp olive oil

¼ tsp black pepper

2 cloves garlic, minced

Combine kale, yams, water, and salt in a skillet; bring to a boil. Cover, reduce heat to medium, and cook 8 minutes. Uncover; cook over high heat until water evaporates. Spoon kale–yam mixture into a bowl; set aside, and keep warm. Heat oil in skillet over medium-low heat. Add pepper and garlic; sauté 3 minutes. Spoon over kale–yam mixture and mix together.

NUTRITIONAL ANALYSIS

Per serving: 155 calories; 2 g fat, 5 g protein, 33 g carbohydrate

Cream of Vegetable Soup
makes 6 servings

1 cup chopped onions

1 clove garlic, crushed

10–12 oz can cream of chicken soup

6 cups cauliflower, cut into small pieces

1 cup chopped celery

1 cup chopped carrots

2 cups chopped broccoli

1 box frozen cut corn

8 cups low-fat chicken broth

1 tsp pepper

optional salt

Steam ½ of the cauliflower, cut into small pieces, and place in small bowl. Heat a large pot, spray with cooking spray, and add onions, celery, and carrots. Cook for 4–5 minutes. dd broccoli and remaining ½ of cauliflower; cook 10 minutes, stirring occasionally. Add pepper, cream of chicken soup, and chicken broth. Bring to a boil and simmer for 20–30 minutes. Use a hand blender to puree the soup completely. Add the bowl of small cauliflower and cut corn to the pot of soup and mix gently. Serve with a sprinkle of parmesan cheese

NUTRITIONAL ANALYSIS

Per serving: 176 calories; 5 g fat, 8 g protein, 29 g carbohydrates

Peasant Salad
makes 4 servings

1 cucumber, cut into small pieces

1 avocado, cut into small pieces

2 tomatoes, cut into small pieces

1 bell pepper (any color) cut into small pieces

1 cup red onion, thinly sliced, separated into rings

1 pound chicken breast, cooked and cut into small pieces

2 low-fat mozzarella cheese sticks, cut into small discs

2 Tbsp red wine vinegar

2 Tbsp olive oil

1½ tsp spices of choice, minced (oregano, basil, thyme, chives, red pepper flakes)

1 tsp, sugar

½ tsp salt

½ tsp black pepper

¼ tsp garlic powder

Combine cucumber, avocado, tomato, bell pepper, onion, chicken, and cheese discs in a large bowl; toss well. Combine vinegar, oil, spices, sugar, salt, pepper, and garlic powder in a small bowl; stir well. Pour over chicken vegetable mixture, tossing to coat. Can be served immediately, or marinated for 30–45 minutes.

NUTRITIONAL ANALYSIS

Per serving: 378 calories; 19 g fat, 36 g protein, 15 g carbohydrate

Homemade Hummus
makes 4 servings

1-15 oz can chick peas (garbanzo beans)

1 Tbsp chopped fresh oregano

2 Tbsp chopped fresh parsley

¼ cup balsamic vinegar

½ Tbsp olive oil

½ tsp salt

½ tsp black pepper

2 cloves garlic, minced

Combine all ingredients in a small bowl and crush with pestle until desired consistency is achieved. Cover and chill.

NUTRITIONAL ANALYSIS

Per serving: 162 calories; 5 g fat, 5 g protein, 25 g carbohydrate

Roasted Potatoes with Carrots and Onions
makes 4 servings

1 lb small red potatoes

1 medium white onion

1 lb carrots

2 cloves garlic

½ Tbsp olive oil

paprika

salt

pepper

Preheat oven to 350°. Wash and dry potatoes. Cut into quarters. Peel carrots and cut into small pieces. Cut onions into small pieces. Evenly distribute potatoes, onions, and carrots in oblong roasting dish. Top mixture and sliced garlic cloves. Season with salt, paprika, and pepper. Drizzle or lightly spray olive oil over the entire mixture. Bake in 350° oven for 40 minutes. Remove from oven when done.

NUTRITIONAL ANALYSIS

Per serving: 177 calories; 2 g fat, 4 g protein, 37 g carbohydrates

Mango Mint Smoothie
makes 1 serving

½ cup fat-free yogurt or 1 scoop protein
   powder or weight-loss shake mix
½ cup frozen mango
3 fresh mint leaves, chopped
6 oz cold water
3–4 ice cubes

Put water and fruit in blender and turn on low. Pour in yogurt or
shake mix and continue blending on low. Add ice cubes slowly as
it blends. Adding more ice will create a lighter and fluffier
smoothie. Add mint leaves. When all ingredients are added, secure
the lid and blend on low for 1–2 minutes, then on high for 30
seconds.

NUTRITIONAL ANALYSIS
Per serving: 180 calories; 0 g fat, 16 g protein, 20 g carbohydrates

Chopped Salad
makes 4 servings

1 cucumber, chopped

1 tomato, diced

1 red bell pepper, chopped

1 cup red onion, chopped

6 oz heart of palm (in water) chopped

1 Tbsp red wine vinegar

1 Tbsp olive oil

1 lemon, juiced

1 anchovy, chopped (optional)

½ tsp salt

½ tsp black pepper

Combine cucumber, tomato, onion, bell pepper, and heart of palm in a large bowl; toss well. Combine vinegar, lemon juice, oil, anchovy, salt and pepper in a small bowl; stir well. Mix everything together in the larger bowl and serve.

NUTRITIONAL ANALYSIS

Per serving: 98 calories; 4 g fat, 4 g protein, 13 g carbohydrates

Black Bean and Corn Salsa
makes 6 servings

2 cups canned yellow corn or frozen cut corn, thawed

½ cup chopped green or red bell pepper

½ cup chopped onion

½ cup chopped fresh cilantro

1 Tbsp chopped fresh jalapeño peppers

15 oz canned black beans, drained

1 can chopped tomatoes

¼ cup red wine vinegar

1 Tbsp olive oil

¼ tsp salt

2 cloves garlic, minced

Combine all ingredients in a large bowl and toss well. Cover and chill.

NUTRITIONAL ANALYSIS

Per serving: 183 calories; 3 g fat, 9 g protein, 33 g carbohydrates

Lime Pistachio Coconut Smoothie
makes 1 serving

1 cup fat-free yogurt or 2 scoops
  protein powder or weight-loss shake mix
½ tsp fat-free pistachio pudding mix
1 Tbsp fresh lime juice
3 drops coconut extract
6 oz cold water
3–4 ice cubes

Put shake mix or yogurt in blender, add the water, and blend on low. Add ice cubes slowly as it blends. Adding more ice will create a lighter and fluffier smoothie. Add pudding mix, lime juice, and extract. When all ingredients are added, secure the lid and blend on low for 1–2 minutes, then on high for 30 seconds.

NUTRITIONAL ANALYSIS

Per serving: 150 calories; 0 g fat, 16 g protein, 16 g carbohydrates

Teriyaki Chicken Kebabs
makes 4 servings

1 lb chicken breast, cut into 24 pieces

1 cup low-sodium teriyaki sauce or marinade

24 pieces cut-up purple onion

24 pieces yellow squash or zucchini

1 Tbsp grated ginger

1 tsp olive oil

3 garlic cloves, minced

24 cherry tomatoes

24 small mushrooms

24 pieces of bell pepper, any color

Combine first 7 ingredients in a large bowl and marinate in refrigerator for 30 minutes. Drain, reserving marinade. Assemble kebabs. Onto 8 wooden skewers, put 3 pieces each, alternating chicken, onion, zucchini, tomatoes, mushrooms, and peppers. Place kebabs on tray and broil or grill for 15–16 minutes. Baste with marinade and turn every 2–3 minutes.

NUTRITIONAL ANALYSIS

Per serving: 391 calories; 5 g fat, 42 g protein, 49 g carbohydrates

Lemon-Garlic Squash
makes 4 servings

2 lb yellow squash and/or zucchini

½ tsp grated lemon zest

2 cloves garlic, chopped

¼ tsp salt

2 small onions

1 tbsp olive oil

Cut the squash into thin, round slices. Steam or microwave until lightly cooked (5–7 minutes). In a large pan or wok, sauté chopped garlic and onions with olive oil for 3–5 minutes. Add salt and lemon zest. Add squash to pan and mix well, cooking over medium-high heat for 1–2 minutes.

NUTRITIONAL ANALYSIS

Per serving: 83 calories; 4 g fat, 2 g protein, 13 g carbohydrates

Egg Salad
makes 6 servings

12 eggs

1 cup diced celery

2 Tbsp chopped green pepper

2 Tbsp chopped onion (optional)

2 Tbsp fat-free mayonnaise

1 Tbsp rice vinegar

1 tsp salt

½ tsp Worcestershire sauce or dijon mustard

½ tsp white pepper

Dash of paprika

4 cups chopped lettuce

Boil the eggs in salt water for 10 minutes, chill. Peel eggs, slice in half, and discard all but 3 yolks. Chop all the egg whites and combine with the 3 yolks. Mix in chopped celery, green pepper, onion; add fat-free mayonnaise, vinegar, salt, Worcestershire sauce or dijon mustard, and pepper. Serve over lettuce. Garnish with paprika.

NUTRITIONAL ANALYSIS

Per serving: 79 calories; 3 g fat, 10 g protein, 3 g carbohydrates

Turkey and Rice Stuffed Peppers
makes 4 servings

4 large green peppers

1 lb lean ground turkey

1 cup chopped onion

½ cup chopped carrots

2 cloves garlic, minced

1 Tbsp olive oil

1 cup cooked brown rice

1 can yellow corn or ½ cup frozen cut corn

½ tsp salt

½ tsp black pepper

8 oz tomato sauce

4 oz low-fat shredded cheese

Cut tops off peppers, wash, and remove seeds. Cook peppers in boiling water for 3 minutes. Remove from water and set aside. Cook turkey over medium-high heat until brown, drain, and set aside. In the same pan, add onion, carrots, garlic, and olive oil; cook for 3 minutes over medium-high heat. Add cooked turkey back to the same pan and mix ingredients well. Add brown rice, corn, and tomato sauce and mix everything together. Fill peppers with mixture and bake at 350° for 20 minutes. Top with cheese and bake another 5 minutes.

NUTRITIONAL ANALYSIS
Per serving: 515 calories; 24 g fat, 41 g protein, 34 g carbohydrates

13

THE LEPTIN LIFESTYLE

Physical Activity

One of the best ways to treat leptin resistance is to ramp up your physical activity. Exercise will have a dramatic effect on lowering your level of leptin resistance. Physical activity reduces leptin resistance, in part, because it makes your muscles metabolically stronger. As the old saying goes, "muscle burns fat."

I recommend that you set a goal of getting at least 60 minutes of physical activity every day. This can be any type of physical activity, from taking a walk to lifting weights. It's helpful and more fun, but of course not mandatory, to do a variety of types of physical activity over the course of a week.

Exercise Versus Physical Activity

Many people don't exercise, because they feel overwhelmed. They make a big deal out of exercise, making sure they have the right clothes, equipment, gym membership, and so on. Most of my patients lose all the weight they want to lose through walking alone. Physical activity is anything you can do to move your body through space. You don't have to join a gym or start a formal exercise program. Anything you can do will help balance your hormones.

I recommend increasing the activities in your life that will help you burn calories. Take a short walk in the morning, go shopping and keep walking, clean the house, or wash the car. It doesn't matter what you do as long as you keep moving. And you don't have to do it all at once, either. Just as I recommend eating small meals frequently throughout the day, I also recommend small bouts of physical activity during the day. This will keep your metabolism supercharged and help your fat-burning machinery go into overdrive.

Physical activity has benefits that go beyond simply burning calories. It's one of the best-known ways to reduce stress. When you have less stress, you'll have less leptin resistance. Cortisol will go down, growth hormone will go up, and insulin resistance will improve.

How Much Physical Activity Is Ideal for Leptin?

I recommend that you get at least one hour per day (or seven hours per week) of physical activity. Why so much? Because this really isn't that much. Back in prehistoric times, humans got hours and hours of physical activity every day as they were out hunting and gathering foods for their very survival. Our delicate hormonal systems are used to a high level of physical activity. Luckily, you don't have to work out for 60 minutes continuously. Still, your ultimate goal should be to get in a total of 60 minutes of physical activity over the course of each and every day.

Many of my patients start off a visit with me by saying that they find it just impossible to get so much exercise. Indeed, if you haven't been doing much lately, this can really seem a big challenge, but almost every one can do this much physical activity. You should start off slow. Even if you begin by doing five minutes per day, you're doing your body good, and you'll feel better.

A good way to start is to take a five-minute walk once a day. Set your watch, walk down the block for two and a half minutes, turn around, and come home. You are done for the day. Over the course of several months, you can gradually increase the amount of time, until you reach your goal. Just don't be overwhelmed, because even a little bit of physical activity is better than none at all.

Water

Keeping the Metabolic Machinery Working

You've heard it before: "drink water to lose weight." Most people know that drinking water is an important part of weight loss, but there's an increasing body of evidence that proper hydration is absolutely necessary for effective weight loss. Diets often fail because of dehydration. If you get dehydrated, your appetite will increase and metabolism will slow. Dehydration slows down metabolism, because all your fat-burning mechanisms are impaired because of lack of water.

As you lose weight, you are losing water, which makes it even more important to get enough water to drink. Losing water is part of losing weight. And for the most part, this is a good thing. If you have excess fat, you have excess water in your body. There's a natural effect of weight loss that tells the kidneys to release more water from the body. But if you don't drink enough—at least 8 glasses each day—your body will become dehydrated.

In the first few weeks of a diet, about 50 percent of the weight you lose is water. Most people find that when they start a diet, they're going to the bathroom all the time. This water loss is a natural and healthy part of weight loss, but if you don't replace the water in your body, you'll become dehydrated. Metabolism will slow and you'll stop losing weight.

Detoxify: Flushing Toxins

We are exposed to chemicals every day. They are everywhere in our environment. You can't avoid them. Pesticides, cleaners, adhesives, preservatives, and other toxins are ubiquitous at home, at school, and in the office. Over the years, toxic substances build up in your fat. As you lose weight and burn fat, the toxins are released into your bloodstream. This can make you feel bad. But drinking plenty of water enables your body to flush the toxins from your system.

Drink Cold Water to Boost Your Metabolism

Studies have shown that drinking ice water will boost your metabolism. Why? Your body has to burn calories to generate heat. When you drink cold water, it cools the body and forces your fat cells to increase heat production in order to keep your body temperature constant. Your fat cells then put their energy into generating heat instead of making you fat.

Dehydration: Subtle or Severe

When you get dehydrated, your metabolism slows, which makes it difficult for your body to burn fat. The signs of dehydration may range from very subtle to severe. They include:

- Constipation
- Decreased sweating
- Decreased urination
- Dizziness on standing
- Dry mouth
- Fatigue
- Headache
- Slow metabolism
- Thirst

Stress Reduction

It is critical for hormonal balance and leptin balance that you reduce your stress. There's nothing worse for your hormones than stress. When it comes to weight gain, stress points just about every hormone in the wrong direction. Stress makes insulin resistance worse. It causes problems with thyroid hormone, growth hormone, and both male and female hormones. Stress is well known for making cortisol levels skyrocket. Stress has the classic double-whammy effect on leptin—increasing leptin resistance while at the same time decreasing leptin production.

Deep-breathing exercises are a terrific way to reduce stress. They help you relax and also increase the amount of oxygen you bring into your body. Oxygen fuels your metabolism. Have you ever seen something burn that doesn't get enough air? It doesn't burn very well. You simply can't burn fat if there's not enough oxygen in your system.

Quality Sleep Is Critical for Leptin Balance

Sleep has a major influence on all your hormones, and leptin is no exception. Good-quality sleep is vital for proper leptin balance. Poor sleep, by contrast, means lower leptin levels and increased appetite. It's been estimated that as many as 35 percent of Americans experience insomnia at one point in their lives, while 15 percent have chronic insomnia. It's more common as you get older, occurring in up to one third of people older than age 65. People with high-stress jobs and lower socioeconomic and education levels have higher rates of insomnia. The vast majority of people with insomnia never receive treatment. Chronic sleep deprivation has been blamed, in part, for America's obesity epidemic. Inadequate sleep has been linked to heart disease, strokes, and cancer. People with chronic insomnia feel bad all the time and in general have poor health.

During sleep, leptin levels rise. If you fail to get enough sleep, or the sleep you do get is of poor quality, your body won't make the leptin it needs. Your fat cells won't be able to communicate with your brain. The misinformed brain will think you're starving. The end result? Weight gain.

When I see patients for sleep problems, my challenge comes from both making a diagnosis and finding a treatment. Sleeping pills such as Ambien, Sonata, and Lunesta are frequently prescribed because they are touted as being "safe and effective." Experts agree, however, that these medications are appropriate for short-term use only. I rarely prescribe sleeping pills for my patients because I feel that it's not actually treating the problem. Sleeping pills are never a long-term solution.

The best way to treat insomnia is to determine the cause and match the treatment to the cause. For most people, there's usually more than one cause—what doctors refer to as multifactorial. Poor sleep hygiene—like watching TV in bed, drinking caffeinated beverages later in the day, or having chaotic bedtimes and wake times—is the most common cause of insomnia. Medical problems like asthma, hyperthyroidism, menopause, congestive heart failure, arthritis, benign prostatic hypertrophy, restless leg syndrome, gastroesophageal reflux disease (GERD), and even depression can all cause insomnia. A study from the National Institute of Mental Health found that as many as 40 percent of people with insomnia have a psychiatric problem. Stress of any type almost always causes sleep disturbances. Many medications affect sleep: often blood pressure medications, antidepressants, anxiety medications, antibiotics. Sleep apnea is a condition that results in poor-quality sleep because of problems breathing during the night. There's also what's called psychophysiological insomnia, a condition in which there's no apparent reason why someone can't fall asleep, stay asleep, or have good-quality sleep.

If you have problems falling asleep or staying asleep, or if you wake up feeling unrested, you should see your physician for an evaluation. Your doctor will take a comprehensive sleep history that will include questions about the pattern and quality or your sleep, falling asleep, staying asleep, dreaming, snoring, waking up, and daytime sleepiness. You should tell your doctor about *all* your symptoms, because any of these may be an important clue. You should keep a record of your sleep—a sleep log—to help your physician make a diagnosis. Insomnia that lasts a week or two is known as "acute insomnia." If it lasts longer than three months, it's called "chronic insomnia."

Treatments for insomnia that don't involve medications are the best way to go. Over the long run, changes in your lifestyle will be much more effective than taking sleeping pills. Besides, lifestyle changes don't have side effects the way sleeping pills do. No matter what the cause, proper sleep hygiene always helps. In my practice I recommend the following sleep hygiene rules:

• Maintain a regular bedtime and wake time, even on the weekends.
• Do not spend more than eight hours in bed each night.
• Make sure you get adequate exposure to light during the day, and avoid bright lights before bedtime.
• Maintain a dark and quiet bedroom.
• Exercise regularly, but don't exercise two hours before bedtime.
• Avoid caffeine, nicotine, and alcohol if you are having problems sleeping.
• Rest and relax for 30 minutes before going to bed.
• Don't take naps.
• Use the bed for sleep only.
• If awake for more than 20 minutes, get up out of the bed and leave the bedroom.

When all else fails, sleep restriction therapy has become a popular way to treat insomnia. Restricting the amount of sleep you have in a night can help improve total sleep time and sleep quality. Studies have shown that sleep restriction therapy takes about eight weeks to work properly. Patients are advised to keep a sleep log for at least two weeks to document sleep time. The amount of time you spend in bed should match your average sleep time. For example, if you sleep about five hours per night, and wake up at 7 a.m., you shouldn't go to bed until 2 a.m. You should try to wake up at the same time every morning. After a few days, start going to bed 15 minutes earlier each night. You should continue to back up your bedtime in 15-minute increments until the proper amount of sleep is achieved. In the beginning, you may feel sleepy during the day, so you should be careful driving or making important decisions. But once you have reset your sleep cycle, your sleep should be of good quality and you should feel well rested during the day.

14

LEPTIN AND YOUR ENVIRONMENT: ENDOCRINE DISRUPTORS

Living a Clean Life in a Leptin-Toxic Environment

Our environment contains so many things that can disrupt both leptin balance and overall hormonal balance. Obviously, it's impossible to avoid them all, however we may try. The key is to minimize your exposure to the substances that are the most harmful to your hormones.

Fast Food

Many experts believe that fast food has addictive properties. Several individuals have even sued the fast food industry, based on the idea that fast food is addictive. Fast food is the ideal food for causing obesity—it's cheap, high in calories, and easy to find. Research on the biological effects of fast food suggests that cravings for these foods aren't just a matter of self-control. The main reward and pleasure center, called the nucleus accumbens, has developed to inspire people to try to find healthy rewards, like sex or food. Addictive drugs such as nicotine, heroin, and cocaine make use of their alluring draw by usurping this center. Eating high-fat food prompts the release of endorphins and dopamine in the nucleus accumbens in just the way that heroin, cocaine, and nicotine do, though in smaller amounts. Such foods create a surge of endorphins and dopamines, which produce feelings of euphoria and pleasure. When someone uses addictive drugs repeatedly, it is believed that they change the brain's chemistry in many ways. High-fat foods can do the same thing.

Foods that are very high in fat and sugar can cause hormonal imbalance in both your brain and your body that's similar to drug addiction. The major difference between a fast-food meal and a regular meal is the total number of calories and fat you get in one sitting. A typical fast food meal can have as many as 2,800 calories—considerably more than what's recommended for an entire day. When you consume this many calories at time, a host of hormones are disrupted. The body simply isn't designed to process so many calories at once.

A study done at the Albert Einstein College of Medicine showed that you can cause disruptions in the leptin system after just a few fatty meals. Another study, at the Rockefeller University in New York, showed that consuming fatty foods can quickly alter the body's hormonal system, causing cravings for more fat. Galanin, a brain hormone that increases appetite and slows down metabolism, increases when you eat high-fat foods. It only takes one high-fat meal to increase galanin production. When children eat fast food, their galanin system can be permanently affected. It is believed that high levels of fats in the blood turn on the genes to produce galanin, resulting in a lifelong addiction to high-fat foods.

Artificial Sweeteners

A lot of controversy continues to swirl around the topics of artificial sweeteners and weight. Our epidemic of childhood obesity has been linked to increased soda consumption. Sodas and sweetened beverages, like sports drinks and flavored teas, have surpassed white bread as the No. 1 source of calories in the American diet. A six-month study done at Children's Hospital in Boston followed two groups of teenagers. The study, published in the journal *Pediatrics,* compared teenagers who substituted sugar-sweetened beverages for bottled water or artificially sweetened drinks with teenagers who continued to consume their usual amount of soda and sweetened drinks. The study found that the teenagers who consumed diet soda lost weight and the teenagers who drank normal soda gained weight. The researchers estimated that one 12-ounce regular soda per day will lead to about 1 pound of weight gain in a month.

Some research even suggests that artificial sweeteners can make you gain weight. Although promoted to help you lose weight, artificial sweeteners like sucralose (Splenda), aspartame (NutraSweet and Equal), or saccharin (Sweet'n Low) may interfere with your efforts to lose weight by confusing your body and disrupting hormonal balance. Critics claim that sugar substitutes sabotage the body's ability to monitor food intake based on a food's taste. This makes people more likely to overindulge in other foods. People who crave sweets turn to artificial sweeteners as a way of helping their sugar cravings, but the substitutes may paradoxically make the cravings worse. Folks take a break by drinking a diet soda, but later in the day they feel ravenous and are craving sweets. Many people find that when they stop using sugar substitutes, their carbohydrate cravings also stop.

A 2004 Purdue University study, published in the *International Journal of Obesity,* showed that artificial sweeteners can cause weight gain in rats. In the study, rats were fed foods with artificial sweeteners. They were compared to a second group of rats that did not receive artificial sweeteners. The rats that consumed artificial sweeteners ate more food overall and gained weight, while the rats not fed artificial sweeteners did not gain weight. The researchers concluded that artificial sweeteners made the rats gain weight because it was tricking the rats' brains, stimulating appetite.

Researchers at the Centre for Advanced Food Studies in Denmark performed a similar study on humans. Two groups of people were fed identical diets in a research setting. The only difference was that one group was served beverages with artificial sweeteners and the other group was served beverages sweetened with real sugar. The people who had artificial sweeteners ate more food than those who had real sugar. Unlike the rats, however, the people who drank beverages with real sugar consumed more calories and gained weight, and the people who drank artificially sweetened drinks lost weight. The overall result of the study was the opposite of the rats study. At the end of 10 weeks, the people who had artificial sweeteners lost about two pounds and the people who had regular sugar drinks gained about three pounds.

These studies show that when you consume artificial sweeteners, your body craves more food. But, of course, humans are not rats. If you can't judge the calorie content of a particular food based on its sweetness, you are more likely to overeat. This is why it is so important to read the labels. The food industry does more to alter food than just adding artificial sweeteners. Even so-called "fat-free" products may cause the same effect. When manufacturers reduce the fat content in foods, they usually increase the sugar to compensate. For example, fat-free ice cream is usually higher in sugar content; sugar-free ice cream is usually higher in fat content. "Sugar free" or "fat free" does not mean "calorie free," and many times the regular counterpart has fewer calories and tastes better.

You'll have a problem if you drink more than one or two artificially sweetened beverages daily. A study presented at the 2005 American Diabetes Association meeting estimates that your risk of being overweight goes up for every diet soda you drink each day. If you consume a lot of artificial sweeteners, you may have increased appetite and will be more likely to overeat other foods. Fortunately, humans have a major advantage over rats: rats can't read labels. You have to read labels to find out how many calories are in the food you eat.

Experts still disagree about the use and effects of artificial sweeteners. My recommendation is to limit your consumption of diet drinks to no more than one or two cans per day. I recommend that you drink mostly water or unsweetened, low-calorie beverages like iced tea or club soda. If you need to sweeten your coffee or tea, use a little bit of real sugar or honey; just don't overdo it. Sodas and other sugary beverages have no nutritional value and should be avoided altogether.

Environmental Toxins

Many compounds in our environment have chemical similarities to the hormone estrogen. These are known as environmental estrogens, or xenoestrogens. Many modern-day chemicals—especially pesticides—have a similar chemical structure to estrogen, and have impacts on leptin, adiponectin, and our overall hormonal balance. Plastic and detergents also contain chemicals similar in structure to estrogen. Environmental estrogens are stored in your fat and released when you lose weight.

It's thought that chemical preservatives may contribute to weight gain by disrupting hormonal balance. Parabens are synthetic preservatives found in shampoos, moisturizers, personal lubricants, make-up foundations, deodorants, and shaving gels; they're also used as food preservatives. One of the parabens—butylparaben— acts like the hormone estrogen. In high levels, this compound can interfere with the body's natural estrogen production, causing hormonal imbalance. These compounds have been thought to cause weight gain and have been linked to breast cancer.

The chemical carbon tetrachloride causes thyroid problems and has been found in drinking water. Polychlorinated biphenyls (PCBs) have also been linked to thyroid dysfunction. The weed killer Roundup, which contains the chemical glyphosate, has been blamed for thyroid problems. Smoking may contribute to thyroid disease because of several toxins, including cadmium, contained in tobacco leaves.

Antibacterial products, from dishwashing liquids to bar soap to toothpaste, contain a chemical called triclosan that is thought to interfere with thyroid hormone metabolism. My recommendation is to avoid antibacterial products. The regular versions of the products do an excellent job of killing microbes, and with no potential risk to your thyroid.

15

MEDICATIONS AND LEPTIN

Many medications affect leptin by helping you lose weight. Some medications can improve leptin resistance, while others can make it worse. There is no perfect medication for leptin. A drug that treats one feature of leptin balance may make another aspect worse. The best strategy is to find a balance between the benefits a medication offers with the risks that it brings. I believe that medications are never a substitute for a healthy diet and regular physical activity.

Diabetes Medications and Leptin

Metformin

One commonly prescribed medication for diabetes is metformin. It decreases the liver's ability to make sugar. Metformin does more than just treat diabetes, though. It decreases insulin resistance and leptin resistance. It increases adiponectin levels as well. Metformin decreases both LDL cholesterol and triglyceride levels.

Metformin has weight loss as a "side effect," which explains some of its effect on leptin resistance. The original, rapid-release formulation of metformin is best for treating leptin resistance. The extended-release formulation is still appropriate for treating leptin resistance and has fewer potential side effects.

Side effects of metformin include diarrhea, nausea, or a queasy stomach. These side effects are usually temporary and go away after two or three days. It's best to start with a low dose and gradually increase over several months. The best dose for improving leptin resistance is 850 mg, taken three times a day. Take metformin with food to lessen side effects.

Thiazolidinediones (TZDs)

TZDs improve both leptin resistance and insulin resistance by stimulating DNA. Patients who take such TZDs as Avandia (rosiglitazone) and Actos (pioglitazone) have lower leptin levels as a result of improved action at its receptor. TZDs also have a potent ability to raise levels of adiponectin. Their cumulative effect is to improve hormone action and overall hormonal balance.

Additional effects of TZDs include lower blood pressure and less inflammation. TZDs lower triglycerides and raise HDL (good) cholesterol. They shift LDL from the dangerous, small dense type to the less dangerous, large fluffy type. TZDs reverse atherosclerosis, cardiovascular disease, and fatty liver disease. TZDs redistribute body fat, decreasing the amount of dangerous visceral fat and increasing the amount of safer subcutaneous fat.

TZDs are known to cause weight gain, but most people gain only a few of pounds; some gain none at all. If you follow the Leptin Boost Diet, you are more likely to lose weight while taking a TZD as part of your regimen. Fluid retention and anemia are other potential side effects of TZDs. The lowest doses (Avandia 2 mg or Actos 15 mg) are best for treating leptin resistance.

Metformin-Thiazolidinedione Combination Tablets

The prescription drug Avandamet combines rosiglitazone and metformin, while Actoplus Met combines pioglitazone and metformin. These medications are ideal for treating insulin resistance and leptin resistance because they work well together. Both are considered "weight neutral" because weight change is not a side effect. Taking the medications as separate pills gives the exact same effect as the combination tablets.

Byetta

Exenatide, brand name Byetta, works by mimicking the actions of the intestinal hormone glucagon-like peptide-1 (GLP-1). It was originally found in the venom of the Gila monster. GLP-1 works by slowing down the digestive system, which helps you to feel full and lose weight. For more information on GLP-1, see Chapter 4. Byetta improves leptin resistance, in part because it has weight loss as a side effect. Nausea is also a possible side effect. A rare side effect is pancreatitis, which is also seen in people who get a Gila monster bite. Byetta is taken as an injection twice a day.

Symlin

Pramlintide, or Symlin, is an injectible diabetes medication that works in conjunction with insulin. Symlin functions by imitating amylin, a pancreatic hormone that regulates blood glucose (for more information, please see Chapter 4). Symlin is not widely used to treat diabetes; endocrinologists, however, believe that this medication holds promise because it causes weight loss. Nausea, vomiting, low blood sugar, and headache are possible side effects of Symlin.

Symlin is starting to gain more attention because scientists have found that when it's combined with leptin, it can have powerful effects on weight loss. Although still in the experimental stages, this drug can potentially help boost the effects of leptin to overcome leptin resistance.

Glyset and Precose

Miglitol (brand name Glyset) and acarbose (Precose) are diabetes medications that work by inhibiting an enzyme in the bowels that helps digest carbohydrates. These medications slow, but do not prevent, the digestion of food. When the rate at which carbohydrates go into the bloodstream is slowed, blood sugars are lowered and there's less insulin resistance and less leptin resistance.

Blood Pressure Medications and Leptin

High blood pressure is a worldwide epidemic. More than 50 million people in the United States (or one in six) have it, but only about half are treated properly. High blood pressure is a major cause of cardiovascular disease, kidney disease, and blindness, and it compounds with leptin resistance and insulin resistance. Experts have noted that at least half of all cases of high blood pressure can be cured with lifestyle changes and weight loss. If you balance your leptin and balance your hormones, you're on your way to having normal blood pressure *without* the use of medications.

Many people with leptin resistance have high blood pressure that requires treatment with medications. Some blood pressure medications can improve leptin resistance, mostly by improving insulin resistance. These medications can reduce the risk of diabetes and cardiovascular disease. Other blood pressure medications can slow metabolism and worsen insulin resistance.

ACE Inhibitors

Angiotensin-converting enzyme, or ACE inhibitors, are good at lowering blood pressure, yet the benefits of these medications go far beyond that effect alone. ACE inhibitors are thought to improve both insulin resistance and leptin resistance. Several studies have shown that ACE inhibitors also reduce the risk of heart attacks, strokes, diabetes, and

ACE INHIBITORS	
Ramapril (Altace)	Benazepril (Lotensin)
Perindopril (Aceon)	Quinapril (Accupril)
Trandolapril (Mavik)	Enalapril (Vasotec)
Lisinopril (Zestril)	Captopril (Capoten)

kidney failure. Side effects include dry cough, high potassium, fatigue, or headache. In rare cases a serious allergic reaction can cause lip and tongue swelling with sudden trouble swallowing or breathing.

Angiotensin Receptor Blockers

ARBs, or angiotensin receptor blockers, work on the same hormone system as ACE inhibitors, but in a slightly different way. The beneficial effects of ARBs are similar to those of ACE inhibitors. Side effects are not typically experienced, but high potassium levels are sometimes seen.

ANGIOTENSIN RECEPTOR BLOCKERS	
Losartan (Cozaar)	Valsartan (Diovan)
Omlesartan (Benicar)	Telmisartan (Micardis)
Candesartan (Atacand)	Eprosartan (Teveten)
Ibesartan (Avapro)	

Coreg

Carvedilol (brand name Coreg) is known as a second-generation beta-blocking medication. Coreg improves insulin resistance and may also help leptin resistance. Other beta-blockers make resistance worse (see below). Side effects include fatigue, slow heart beat, or difficulty breathing.

Diuretics

Potassium is a mineral that's critical for hormonal balance. Low potassium causes insulin resistance and leptin resistance. Potassium-sparing diuretics are mild diuretics that lower blood pressure while raising potassium levels. Side effects can include liver problems or potassium that goes too high.

POTASSIUM-SPARING DIURETICS	
Spironolactone (Aldactone)	Triamterine (Dyrenium)
Amilioride (Midamor)	Eplerenone (Inspra)

Cholesterol (Lipid) Medications and Leptin

Lipid (cholesterol and triglyceride) problems are extremely common when you have leptin resistance. The classic pattern that's seen in patients with leptin resistance is elevated levels of LDL (bad) cholesterol and triglycerides, accompanied by a reduced level of HDL (good) cholesterol. It's not surprising, therefore, that many people with leptin resistance end up taking medications to lower bad cholesterol, lower triglycerides, or raise good cholesterol. Frequently, after weight loss is achieved, medications can be reduced or even discontinued.

Statins

A class of drugs known as statins has proven to be highly effective in lowering cholesterol in patients with leptin resistance. Statins work by inhibiting the enzyme HMG CoA reductase, which is needed to produce bad cholesterol. The trouble is, the amount of LDL cholesterol is not always the problem in leptin resistance. Leptin resistance decreases the quality of LDL, shifting it to the dangerous, small dense type. Statins help because they improve the quality of LDL from the dangerous, small dense type that can more easily lodge in blood vessels to the less dangerous, large fluffy type.

Statins have antioxidant and anti-inflammatory properties that decrease leptin resistance. Statins reduce the risk of cardiovascular disease and can even reverse it. This effect seems to go beyond what we would expect from simply lowering cholesterol.

Many recent studies have confirmed the long-term benefits of statin medications. Statins are being prescribed more and more commonly, and in higher doses than ever before.

Doctors and researchers have vigorously debated which statin is best. Some statin manufacturers make claims based on research studies alone, although not all statin medications have been tested in precisely the same way. Their claims may simply be based on the testing that was done, and may not prove a true difference in the medication. Although dosing may vary, most experts agree that all statin medications are basically the same.

The most common side effect of statin medications is muscle problems. These can range from mild muscle aches to more severe muscle problems. Because statins have such tremendous health benefits, most physicians now recommend that you continue taking it if it is causing only mild muscle pain. Inflammation of the liver is an infrequent side effect. Your doctor will need to monitor liver tests periodically.

STATIN MEDICATIONS AND STARTING DOSE	
Atorvastatin (Lipitor) (10 mg)	Fluvastatin (Lescol) (40 mg)
Pravastatin (Pravachol) (20 mg)	Lovastatin (Mevacor) (40 mg)
Simvistatin (Zocor) (20 mg)	Rosuvastatin (Crestor) (5 mg)

Fibrates

These drugs, called fibrates, are derivatives of a compound known as fibric acid. Fenofibrate and an older medication, gemfibrozil (Lopid), are chemically similar to the thiazolidinedione medications Avandia and Actos. Fibrates are a perfect choice for leptin resistance because they lower triglycerides and LDL cholesterol while raising HDL cholesterol. Side effects are uncommon, but liver problems or muscle problems can occur.

FIBRATES	
Tricor (fenofibrate)	Triglide (fenofibrate)
Lofibra (fenofibrate)	Lopid (gemfibrozil)
Antara (fenofibrate)	

Niaspan

The medication Niaspan is an extended-release formulation of niacin, also known as nicotinic acid or vitamin B3. Niacin treats the multiple lipid abnormalities associated with leptin resistance.

Niaspan works to lower triglycerides and LDL cholesterol and to raise HDL cholesterol. Side effects include flushing, tingling, or redness of the skin. To minimize side effects, you should start with a low dose of Niaspan and gradually increase the dose over several months. The flushing can also be reduced by taking an aspirin with a full glass of water one hour before taking Niaspan. A concern with Niaspan and all products that contain niacin is that it can worsen insulin resistance and leptin resistance. For most people, this potential problem never occurs and niacin can be useful for an overall plan of health and wellness. Short-acting niacin is available as a nutritional supplement without a prescription, but it should be taken only under medical supervision.

Omacor

The medication Omacor is a prescription form of the omega-3 fatty acids that may improve leptin resistance. It is approved by the Food and Drug Administration to treat high triglycerides, but it also works to improve insulin resistance and helps raise leptin and adiponectin levels. The prescription formulation is better than over-the-counter preparations because it is more pure and thus more potent.

Other Medications That Help Leptin

A myriad of medications have an effect on leptin, helping with weight loss. This list continues to grow. Listed below are merely a few of the many medications that have been thought to be beneficial for achieving leptin balance.

Antidepressants

All antidepressants work by altering the brain hormones serotonin, norepinephrine, and dopamine. These potent chemicals work in the same regions of the brain as leptin. While some antidepressants tend to cause weight gain, others may cause weight loss. It is thought that antidepressants can improve leptin resistance and insulin resistance through causing weight loss. But treating depression can also lower cortisol levels, which in turn can improve leptin resistance as well.

Effexor and Cymbalta are very similar to the weight-loss medication Meridia. These medications decrease appetite and help with weight loss, yet the effect is mild. They can cause insomnia, high blood pressure, and rapid heartbeat. Wellbutrin is another antidepressant that induces mild weight loss through the brain hormone dopamine. Side effects include insomnia, agitation, and even seizures.

Topiramate (Topamax) and Zonisamide (Zonegran)

Topamax and Zonegran are traditionally used to treat seizures and migraine headaches. They work by decreasing GABA levels. They also help with weight loss and can decrease appetite and stop overeating. These medications are very useful in reducing binge eating and overeating at night. Side effects include sedation and kidney stones, memory problems, and tingling of the hands.

Rimonabant (Acomplia)

The drug rimonabant works by blocking substances in the brain known as endocannabinoids. It blocks the brain's ability to receive hunger signals. Rimonabant improves leptin resistance because it helps people with food cravings reduce their overeating. The endocannabinoid system is a system of natural brain peptides that regulates metabolism, appetite, and energy levels. Nausea, vomiting and depression are possible side effects of rimonabant.

Testosterone Replacement Therapy (for Men Only)

Men with leptin resistance are at high risk for having low testosterone levels. The goal of treating testosterone deficiency is to alleviate the symptoms of hypogonadism and to bring testosterone levels into the normal range. Testosterone replacement therapy improves leptin action and improves metabolism. TRT comes in a variety of formulations. Testosterone pills should *not* be used in men, because this form of TRT causes liver toxicity.

TESTOSTERONE REPLACEMENT THERAPIES	
Androgel (gel)	Striant (buccal tablet)
Testim (gel)	Testosterone cypionate (injection)
Testoderm (patch)	Testosterone enanthate (injection)
Androderm (patch)	

Birth Control Pills (for Women Only)

The tried-and-true birth control pill used by women can lower excess male hormones, which in turn can improve leptin resistance. Birth control pills contain synthetic versions of the hormones estrogen and progesterone. The amount of estrogen and the type of progesterone are what make each pill different. Synthetic progesterone, known as progestin, can stimulate the androgen receptor, leading to leptin problems. I recommend birth control pills that contain the progestins norgestimate, desogestrel, or drospirenone. These progestins are the best ones for achieving overall leptin balance. The progestins norethindrone, levonorgestrel, and norgestrel can worsen leptin resistance.

Side effects of birth control pills include headaches, nausea, breast tenderness, acne, depression, and PMS. While birth control pills containing high doses of estrogen may also cause weight gain, the medium- and low-dose pills do not. Life-threatening blood clots, heart attacks, and strokes are also a risk with birth control pills. The

BEST BIRTH CONTROL PILLS FOR LEPTIN	
Apri	Othocept
Desogen	Yasmin
Ortho-Cyclin	Yaz
Ortho Tri-Cyclen	

risk is highest if you smoke cigarettes. Women who smoke should never use birth control pills.

Hormone Replacement Therapy (for Women Only)

Estrogen replacement therapy (ERT) or hormone replacement therapy (HRT) can improve leptin resistance and raise adiponectin levels. HRT is not for everyone, and its use in the treatment of leptin problems is considered controversial. If you use estrogen, I recommend that you use products that contain *estradiol*. This is the healthiest type of estrogen that's best for improving leptin resistance. Estradiol is the main ingredient in many common forms of prescription HRT products. The estradiol in prescription formulations is derived from plants and is exactly the same as the estradiol made by your body, so it's considered natural and bioidentical.

Side effects of HRT include breast tenderness, nausea, and swelling. HRTs also have an increased risk of heart attacks, strokes, blood clots, gall bladder problems, and breast cancer. To prevent cancer of the uterus, progesterone medications must be taken with HRT, unless you've had a hysterectomy. The best progesterone is a natural form of progesterone called Prometrium. Synthetic progesterone medications can worsen leptin resistance (see below). As with many other medications, HRT comes with both risks and benefits. If you're going to take it, you and your doctor will need to work together to make sure that the benefits outweigh any risks.

HRT PRODUCTS THAT CONTAIN ESTRADIOL	
Estrace	Prefest
Activella	CombiPatch
FemHRT	

Prescription B-Vitamins

Foltx is a prescription formulation of three vitamins—folate, vitamin B6, and vitamin B12. Metanx is another prescription vitamin medication that contains the active forms of these vitamins—methylfolate, pyridoxal phosphate, and methylcobalamin. B-vitamins lower levels of the toxic amino acid called homocysteine, and they're thought to help reduce the risk of cardiovascular disease, Alzheimer's disease, kidney problems, and certain types of anemia.

Medications That Disrupt Leptin Balance

For you to achieve hormonal balance, it's important to avoid, whenever possible, any and all medications that can worsen leptin resistance. Medications can increase leptin resistance for a variety of reasons.

Antidepressants

Medications that treat depression have a variable effect on weight. In the previous section, I discussed antidepressants that help with weight loss and can improve leptin resistance. Some antidepressants, however, increase appetite and cause significant weight gain. Older antidepressants, such as Elavil and Pamelor, frequently cause massive weight gain. Mirtazapine (Remeron) can also boost appetite and so cause weight gain. SSRIs, or selective serotonin reuptake inhibitors, such as Prozac, Lexapro, Celexa, Zoloft, and Paxil, have variable effects on weight. In my experience, most people lose weight during the first six months they take the medication and then gain it back during the next six months.

Antipsychotic Medications

Medications to treat psychosis have been around since the 1950s. These medications work through the brain hormone dopamine. They have greatly improved the outlook for many patients with mental illness. Antipsychotic drugs are often very effective in treating symptoms of schizophrenia, like hallucinations and bizarre

MEDICATIONS HARMFUL TO LEPTIN BALANCE

Antidepressants: Amitriptyline (Elavil), nortriptyline (Pamelor, Aventyl), mirtazapine (Remeron)

Antipsychotic medications: Olanzapine (Zyprexa), Risperidone (Risperdal), Quetiapine (Seroquel), haloperidol (Haldol), chlorpromazine (Thorazine)

Antiseizure medications: Carbamazepine (Tegretol), Gabapentin (Neurontin)

Beta-blockers: Propanolol (Inderal), Metoprolol (Toprol), Atenolol (Tenormin)

Corticosteroids: (glucocorticoids—prednisone, hydrocortisone, dexamethasone, methylprednisolone)

Diuretics: Furosemide (Lasix), Torsemide (Demadex), Bumetanide (Bumex), Indapamide (Lozol), and Hydrochlorothiazide (HCTZ, Microzide, Hydrodiuril), and Chlorothiazide (Diuril)

HIV/AIDS medications: Amprenavir (Agenerase), tipranavir (Aptivus), nelfinavir (Viracept), ritonavir (Norvir), saquinavir (Invirase, Fortovase), tipranavir (Aptivus), indinavir (Crixivan), fosamprenavir (Lexiva), atazanavir (Reyataz), darunavir (Prezista)

Sedating antihistamines: Diphenhydramine, Doxylamine

Sulfonylureas: Glyburide (DiaBeta), Glipizide (Glucotrol), Glimepiride (Amaryl)

Synthetic progestins: Medroxyprogesterone (Provera), Norethindrone acetate (Aygestin), Megestrol (Megace), Micronor, Nor-QD, Ovrette, Depo-Provera, Norplant; norgestrel and norethindrone (found in birth control pills)

---

thoughts. The medications are also used to treat a variety of other conditions, such as depression, anxiety, chronic pain, and obsessive-compulsive disorder. The older antipsychotics medications, like Haldol or Thorazine, aren't used much anymore because they have been supplanted by a new generation of more effective medications. The newer medicines include Zyprexa, Seroquel, and Risperdal. These drugs can cause massive weight gain, leptin resistance, insulin resistance, and diabetes. Although great for treating mental illness, the new antipsychotics can destroy hormonal balance. Only one drug in this class, aripiprazole (Abilify), does not seem to make people gain weight. It tends to cause insomnia, however, which limits its use.

Antiseizure Medications

Like antidepressants, antiseizure medications can have a variable effect on your weight. In the previous section I discussed Topamax and Zonegran and their potent ability to decrease appetite. On the other end of the scale, Tegretol, Depakote, Dilantin, and Neurontin are seizure medications that typically make people gain weight. Antiseizure medications affect your weight through the GABA system.

Beta-Blockers

Medications for beta-blocking are commonly used to treat such complications of leptin resistance as high blood pressure and congestive heart failure. Inderal, Toprol, and Tenormin are the most commonly used beta-blockers. An unfortunate side effect is slowing of the metabolism. On average, these medications will make you gain about a half pound per month, but some people gain more weight than that. Another problem is that these medications cause elevated levels of the hormone norepinephrine, which can worsen leptin resistance and insulin resistance and can decrease adiponectin levels. Beta-blocking medications increase triglyceride levels and lower HDL (good) cholesterol levels.

Coreg is a second-generation beta-blocker that does not seem to have these problems. Coreg is listed in the section above as being beneficial to leptin. Its effects on leptin resistance, insulin resistance, adiponectin, triglycerides, and HDL cholesterol are the opposite of traditional beta-blocking medications.

Corticosteroids

Also known as glucocorticoids, corticosteroids worsen leptin resistance because they're versions of the hormone cortisol. This class of drugs includes prednisone, dexamethasone, methylprednisolone, and hydrocortisone. Excessive cortisol causes severe leptin resistance and insulin resistance, as well as massive weight gain and muscle loss. These medications can also cause cardiovascular disease, high blood pressure, and diabetes—the very ailments that are linked to leptin resistance.

Diuretics

Also known as "water pills," diuretics work by stimulating the kidneys. Common brands include Lasix, Demadex, Bumex, Lozol, Diuril, and Hydrochlorothiazide. They work by making the kidneys release excess water, but they also cause the body to lose important minerals, such as potassium, magnesium, chromium, and selenium. The most potent effect is on potassium, so virtually all people who take diuretic medications must also take a potassium supplement. It's important to avoid low potassium, because this can cause insulin resistance, which leads to leptin resistance and sets off a cascade of hormonal imbalance. If you have taken diuretic medications for a prolonged period, your body may be deficient in many trace minerals. A class of diuretics, known as potassium-sparing diuretics, is listed in the section above; these can be beneficial for maintaining leptin balance.

HIV/AIDS Medications

A class of HIV/AIDS drugs, called protease inhibitors, causes a condition known as HIV lipodystrophy. Lipodystrophy results in a shifting of the body fat, with loss of healthy fat and an increase in the unhealthy visceral fat. People with lipodystrophy have leptin resistance and insulin resistance, and also have higher blood sugar and triglyceride levels but lower HDL (good) cholesterol levels. Patients with lipodystrophy also have very low levels of adiponectin. Some research has shown that experimental leptin and adiponectin medications may block these side effects.

Sedating Antihistamines

Older antihistamines like diphenhydramine and doxylamine, which are found in many over-the-counter sleeping pills and cold remedies, can cause weight gain and worsen leptin resistance.

Sulfonylureas

Many people with leptin resistance take sulfonylurea medications because they are used to treat type 2 diabetes. Unfortunately, in the long run, these medications only put a Band-Aid on the problem. They work by stimulating the pancreas to produce more insulin, thus lowering blood sugar. Sulfonylureas cause weight gain, therefore worsening leptin resistance.

Synthetic Progestins

Progestins are medications that resemble the female hormone progesterone. Synthetic progestins don't really work exactly like progesterone, and can have effects like male hormones and also cause insulin problems. The androgenic progestins levonorgestrel, norgestrel, and norethindrone can increase leptin and insulin resistance, raise blood sugar, and cause both weight gain and depression.

16

VITAMINS, MINERALS, AND SUPPLEMENTS

Many vitamins, minerals, and nutritional supplements on the market today are reported to affect leptin or other hormones involved in appetite and body weight. Nutritional supplements are not under as strict regulation as traditional medications. The quality control is highly variable. Many nutritional supplements have not been properly tested. This is not to put down supplements completely, for many of them show promise. But my warning is to learn what you're getting. Many nutritional supplements are derived from plants, but some are hormone preparations made from ground animal glands or brains. The labels can be disguised (*bovine* means cow, *porcine* means pig) and you may end up buying something that is indeed "natural" but not necessarily helpful. Vitamins and minerals can also come from the foods we eat. You don't always have to "pop a pill."

Zinc

The most important nutrient related to leptin production is zinc. People deficient in zinc have very low leptin levels. You can get zinc deficiency from a poor diet, heavy alcohol use, digestive problems, or chronic kidney disease, and even from diuretic medications. Symptoms of zinc deficiency include dry skin, hair loss, diarrhea, emotional problems, infections, and fatigue. Zinc also has an important function in regulating your taste buds. Foods high in zinc include oysters, fish, turkey, sunflower seeds, beef, wheat germ, lima beans, and dairy products.

Chromium

For insulin to work properly it must have access to chromium. If insulin doesn't work right, neither does leptin. You only need a small amount of chromium in your diet, but if you develop chromium deficiency you'll have both insulin resistance and leptin resistance. Doctors usually don't do blood tests for chromium deficiency because the tests are not accurate. If you have leptin resistance, you're more likely to lose excess chromium in your urine and sweat.

Foods high in chromium include mushrooms, wheat germ, brewer's yeast, beef, broccoli, chicken, shellfish, corn, whole grains, and fruit. Chromium supplements (500–1,000 mcg daily) can also improve leptin and insulin resistance.

Selenium

The antioxidant selenium reduces inflammation and decreases leptin resistance. In addition, selenium has a second role: besides its antioxidizing properties, it helps produce the active form of thyroid hormone known as T3. Selenium deficiency reduces levels of active thyroid hormone by preventing its conversion from the inactive form, or T4. Although selenium supplements are available from most health food stores, I recommend that you increase your consumption of this mineral by eating the proper foods. Foods high in selenium include mushrooms, whole grains, wheat germ, oats, tuna, halibut, and sunflower seeds. Too much selenium, however, can be as damaging as too little. Among the side effects of too much selenium are diarrhea, belly pain, and nerve problems. If you do take supplements, 50 mcg a day is the recommended dose.

Calcium

Studies have also shown that calcium, especially in the form of low-fat dairy products, will accelerate weight loss. It's thought that calcium speeds up fat-burning enzymes in the body. I recommend a minimum of 1,000–1,500 mg of calcium daily in the food you eat or in supplements, or both. Calcium should be consumed over the course of the day, not all at once, and with lots of water.

Magnesium

The mineral magnesium is important for the functioning of many hormones. Leptin resistance can cause your body to become deficient in magnesium. Diuretic medications and heavy alcohol use can also cause magnesium deficiency. Symptoms of magnesium deficiency include fatigue, insomnia, anxiety, muscle weakness, aches and pains, leg cramps or restless legs, hearing loss, constipation, and attention and memory problems. Some people believe that magnesium has a calming effect on the body. The best way to get magnesium is by eating more magnesium-rich foods like tofu, spinach, broccoli, Swiss chard, beans, tomatoes, turnip greens, pumpkin seeds, okra, and lentils. Low-fat dairy products are also a good source of magnesium. Magnesium supplements come in the form of magnesium oxide or magnesium hydroxide and are sold as antacids and laxatives. I don't usually recommend magnesium supplements, except in more severe cases.

B-Vitamins: Folate, B6, and B12

B-vitamins prevent complications of leptin resistance, including blood clots and cardiovascular disease. They help the body break down the toxic substance homocysteine.

One of the B-vitamins, folic acid is found in green leafy vegetables, avocados, whole grains, oranges, bananas, and nuts. Folic acid supplements of 1,000 micrograms (1 milligram, or mg) can also be helpful.

Vitamin C

A powerful antioxidant that boosts the immune system, good old vitamin C fights cancer and prevents cardiovascular disease. It's also an important component of collagen, a vital structural material in the body. When someone has vitamin C deficiency, or scurvy, the body's structural material weakens. Weakening occurs of muscle, skin, bone, and other tissues. Symptoms of vitamin C deficiency include weakness, fatigue, thin skin, easy bruising, and bleeding gums. In today's day and age you would think scurvy is rare, suffered only by pirates, but it is not. I have treated hundreds of patients with vitamin C deficiency, most of whom were amazed to find out what was causing their symptoms. The best way to get vitamin C is through citrus fruits, like oranges, tangerines, grapefruit, lemons, and limes. Broccoli, strawberries, and other vegetables are also great sources of vitamin C. If you take a supplement, the standard dose is 500–1,000 mg daily.

Vitamin D

Deficiency of vitamin D is a major cause of bone and muscle problems in the United States. Vitamin D is actually a steroid hormone, one that allows your intestines to absorb calcium and other nutrients. Most people don't get enough vitamin D from sunlight and dairy products alone. Vitamin D deficiency can cause leptin problems as well as bone pain and fatigue. The recommended daily dose is 800–1,000 IU (international units) of vitamin D.

Omega-3

Supplements containing omega-3 fatty acids can improve leptin resistance. You can get omega-3 from eating cold-water fish. Supplements are available as a prescription formulation called Omacor as well as over-the-counter products.

Caffeine

When it comes to leptin, caffeine is a controversial topic. Caffeine is a common ingredient in many over-the-counter weight-loss products, but the research that supports its effectiveness is marginal at best. Some research suggests that caffeine actually increases appetite. Certain studies have shown that people who drink more coffee have a decreased risk of getting diabetes, but no one knows if this effect is from the caffeine or some other substance in the coffee.

Some experts blame caffeine for contributing to weight gain and obesity. Coffee and caffeine intake can worsen physical, mental, and emotional stress, leading to increased levels of the stress hormone cortisol. A good relationship is observed between chronically elevated levels of cortisol and weight gain.

My opinion is that drinking coffee, tea, or other caffeinated beverages in moderation has very little effect on overall hormonal balance.

Cinnamon

The simple spice cinnamon can reduce blood sugar levels and lead to improved leptin resistance and insulin resistance. Cinnamon has insulin-like properties that can lower blood sugar and may perhaps prevent diabetes. The active ingredient is found in powdered cinnamon, not cinnamon oil. The best way to get cinnamon is to add about ½ teaspoon per day to foods like coffee, yogurt, or cereal.

Garlic

With both antioxidant and anti-inflammatory properties, garlic can improve leptin resistance. It can also lower cholesterol levels. To get a good effect from the odorous bulb, you have to consume several large cloves every day. Garlic pills are an odorless, tasteless formulation that allows you to get enough while avoiding garlic breath.

Fiber

Leptin resistance is improved by fiber, for several reasons. Fiber adds bulk and volume to your meals without adding calories. It helps you feel satisfied and stimulates release of the appetite-suppressing hormones adiponectin and cholecystokinin, while lowering insulin and ghrelin levels. Fiber lowers the glycemic index and glycemic load of foods, which slows the rate at which sugar hits your bloodstream. Vegetables, fruits, and whole grains are the best sources of fiber. The Leptin Boost Diet emphasizes foods that are high in fiber. High-fiber cereals and over-the-counter fiber supplements such as Benefiber, Metamucil, and Citrucel are another way to increase fiber in your diet.

Soy Menopause Supplements

Natural menopause products contain compounds called isoflavones. These compounds are derived from soybeans and work because they imitate healthy estrogens. These compounds are similar to estrogen and, for the most part, seem to be healthy. Still, much controversy swirls around these products. Concentrations of isoflavones can vary tremendously from brand to brand and pill to pill. The results of studies of these products has noted tremendous variability in their effectiveness.

Chocolate

I'm happy to report that chocolate contains over 300 active ingredients, many of which are thought to have health-promoting properties. Chocolate contains antioxidants that help prevent cardiovascular disease and cancer. The antioxidants in chocolate are called flavonoids and polyphenols, and are the same compounds found in red wine, green tea, fruits, and vegetables. Chocolate does contain fat, but the fat in dark chocolate is a healthy type of fat. It's mostly a saturated vegetable fat, similar to olive and canola oils. Chocolate contains important vitamins and nutrients such as magnesium, iron, calcium, phosphorus, potassium, and vitamins A, C, D, and E.

Chocolate contains small amounts of a chemical called phenylethylamine (PEA) that's known as a "happy" brain chemical. PEA is highest during times of joy and love. Chocolate also contains theobromine, which has the same effect on the brain as some antidepressants, offering a rush of serotonin and a calming influence. Chocolate can boost endorphin levels in the brain. Endorphins are brain chemicals that induce a feeling of happiness and elation. These chemicals are responsible for what's sometimes called "runners high," that feeling of calmness and euphoria felt during peak physical exertion. Chocolate contains acylethanolamines, chemicals that may have a similar effect on the brain as marijuana, causing calmness and happiness.

For all these reasons, I recommend eating chocolate. But not all chocolate is the same. The healthiest chocolate is dark chocolate. I recommend eating chocolate that has 70 percent cocoa or higher. Just one or two small squares each day is enough.

PART IV

USEFUL INFORMATION

FOOD DIARY

Day:
- [ ] Monday
- [ ] Tuesday
- [ ] Wednesday
- [ ] Thursday
- [ ] Friday
- [ ] Saturday
- [ ] Sunday

Date:

Notes:

Meal: Breakfast

Breakfast Time:

Food & Beverage: Serving Size/Exchanges: Calories:

Caloric Intake

Total: _____   Goal: _____

Meal: Mid-morning Snack

Mid-morning Snack Time:

Food & Beverage: Serving Size/Exchanges: Calories:

Caloric Intake

Total: _____   Goal: _____

Meal: Lunch

Lunch Time:

Food & Beverage: Serving Size/Exchanges: Calories:

Caloric Intake

Total: _____   Goal: _____

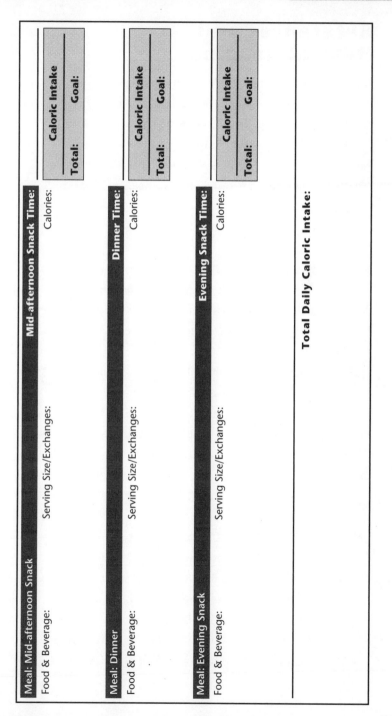

Meal: Mid-afternoon Snack

Mid-afternoon Snack Time:

Food & Beverage: Serving Size/Exchanges: Calories:

Caloric Intake

Total: Goal:

Meal: Dinner

Dinner Time:

Food & Beverage: Serving Size/Exchanges: Calories:

Caloric Intake

Total: Goal:

Meal: Evening Snack

Evening Snack Time:

Food & Beverage: Serving Size/Exchanges: Calories:

Caloric Intake

Total: Goal:

Total Daily Caloric Intake:

References and Helpful Reading

American Association of Clinical Endocrinologists Hypertension Task Force. 2006. AACE Guidelines for Clinical Practice for the Diagnosis and Treatment of Hypertension. *Endocrine Practice* 12, no. 2 (March/April).

American Association of Clinical Endocrinologists/American Diabetes Association Task Force on Inpatient Diabetes. 2006. AACE and ADA Consensus Statement on Inpatient Diabetes and Glycemic Control. *Endocrine Practice* 12. Suppl. no. 3 (July/August).

Ahima, R. S., and J. S. Flier. 2000. Adipose Tissue as an Endocrine Organ. *Trends in Endocrinology and Metabolism* 11:327–32.

Arner, P. 2006. Visfatin: A True or False Trail to Type 2 Diabetes Mellitus. *Journal of Clinical Endocrinology and Metabolism* 91:28–30.

Badman, M. K., and J. S. Flier. 2005. The Gut and Energy Balance: Visceral Allies in the Obesity Wars. *Science Magazine* 307: 1909–14.

Banerjee, R. R., and M. A. Lazar. 2003. Resistin: Molecular History and Prognosis. *Journal of Molecular Medicine* 81:218–26.

Banerjee, R. R., S. M. Rangwala, J. S. Shapiro, A. S. Rich, B. Rhoades, Y. Qi, J. Wang, et al. 2004. Regulation of Fasted Blood Glucose by Resistin. *Science Magazine* 303:1195–98.

Belanger, C. V. Luu-The, P. Dupont, and A. Tchernof. 2002. Adipose Tissue Intracrinology: Potential Importance of Local Androgen/Estrogen Metabolism in the Regulation of Adiposity. *Hormone Metabolism Research* 34:737–45.

Berg, A. H., T. Combs, X. Du, M. Brownlee, and P. E. Scherer. 2001. The Adipocyte-Secreted Protein Acrp30 Enhances Hepatic Insulin Action. *Nature Medicine* 7:947–53.

Berg, A. H., Y. Lin, M. P. Lisanti, and P. E. Scherer. 2004.
Adipocyte Differentiation Induces Dynamic Changes in NF-
kappaβ Expression and Activity. *American Journal of
Physiology, Endocrinology and Metabolism* 287:E1178–88.

Bjorbaek, C. and B. B. Kahn. 2004. Leptin Signaling in the Central
Nervous System and the Periphery. *Recent Progress in Hormone
Research* 59:305–31.

Bobbert, T., H. Rochlitz, U. Wegewitz, S. Akpulat, K. Mai, M. O.
Weickert, M. Mohlig, A. F. Pfeiffer, and J. Spranger. 2005.
Changes of Adiponectin Oligomer Composition by Moderate
Weight Reduction. *Diabetes* 54:2712–19.

Campfield, L. A., F. J. Smith, Y. Guisez, et al. 1998. Recombinant
Mouse OB Protein: Evidence for a Peripheral Signal Linking
Adiposity and Central Neural Networks. *Science Magazine* 269:
546–49.

Chan, J. L., K. Heist, A. DePaoli, J. D. Veldhuis, and C. S.
Mantzoros. 2003. The Role of Falling Leptin Levels in the
Neuroendocrine and Metabolic Adaptation to Short-term
Starvation in Healthy Men. *Journal of Clinical Investigation*
111:1409–21.

Chandran, M., S. A. Phillips, T. Ciaraldi, and R. R. Henry. 2003.
Adiponectin: More Than Just Another Fat Cell Hormone?
Diabetes Care 26:2442–50.

Chen, H., O. Charlat, L. A. Tartaglia, E. A. Woolf, W. Weng, S. J.
Ellis, N. D. Lakey, et al. 1996. Evidence That the Diabetes Gene
Encodes the Leptin Receptor: Identification of a Mutation in
the Leptin Receptor Gene in db/db Mice. *Cell* 84:491–95.

Cianflone, K., M. Maslowska, and A. D. Sniderman. 1999. Acyla-
tion Stimulating Protein (ASP), an Adipocyte Autocrine: New
Directions. *Seminars in Cell & Developmental Biology* 10:31–41.

Cock, T. A., and J. Auwerx. 2003. Leptin: Cutting the Fat Off the
Bone. *The Lancet* 362:1572–74.

Coleman, D. L. 1973. Effects of Parabiosis of Obese with Diabetes and Normal Mice. *Diabetologia* 9:294–98.

Combs, T. P., A. H. Berg, S. Obici, P. E. Scherer, and L. Rossetti. 2001. Endogenous Glucose Production is Inhibited by the Adipose-Derived Protein Acrp30. *Journal of Clinical Investigation* 108:1875–81.

Combs, T. P., U. B. Pajvani, A. H. Berg, Y. Lin, L. A. Jelicks, M. Laplante, A. R. Nawrocki, et al. 2004. A Transgenic Mouse with a Deletion in the Collagenous Domain of Adiponectin Displays Elevated Circulating Adiponectin and Improved Insulin Sensitivity. *Endocrinology* 145:367–83.

Combs, T. P., J. A. Wagner, J. Berger, T. Doebber, W. J. Wang, B. B. Zhang, M. Tanen, et al. 2002. Induction of Adipocyte Complement-Related Protein of 30 Kilodaltons by PPAR Famma Agonists: A Potential Mechanism of Insulin Sensitization. *Endocrinology* 143:998–1007.

Cook, K. S., H. Y. Min, D. Johnson, R. J. Chaplinsky, J. S. Flier, C. R. Hunt, and B. M. Spiegelman. 1987. Adipsin: A Circulating Serine Protease Homolog Secreted by Adipose Tissue and Sciatic Nerve. *Science Magazine* 237:402–405.

Degawa-Yamauchi, M., K. A. Moss, J. E. Bovenkerk, S. S. Shankar, C. L. Morrison, C. J. Lelliott, A. Vidal-Puig, R. Jones, and R. V. Considine. 2005. Regulation of Adiponectin Expression in Human Adipocytes: Effects of Adiposity, Glucocorticoids, and Tumor Necrosis Factor-alpha. *Obesity* 13:662–69.

Dejager, S., A. LeBeaut, A. Couturier, and A. Schweizer. 2006. Sustained Reduction in HbA1c During One-year Treatment with Galvus in Patients with Type 2 Diabetes (T2DM). Paper presented at the meeting of the American Diabetes Association, Washington, DC.

Diez, J. J., and P. Iglesias. 2003. The Role of the Novel Adipocyte-Derived Hormone Adiponectin in Human Disease. *European Journal of Endocrinology* 148:293–300.

Ebbeling, C. B., H. A. Feldman, S. K. Osganian, V. R. Chomitz, S. J. Ellenbogen, and D. S. Ludwig. 2006. Effects of Decreasing Sugar-Sweetened Beverage Consumption on Body Weight in Adolescents: A Randomized, Controlled Pilot Study. *Pediatrics* 117:673–80.

Fisher, F. F., M. E. Trujillo, W. Hanif, A. H. Barnett, P. G. McTernan, P. E. Scherer, and S. Kumar. 2005. Serum High Molecular Weight Complex of Adiponectin Correlates Better with Glucose Tolerance Than Total Serum Adiponectin in Indo-Asian Males. *Diabetologia* 48:1084–87.

Flier, J. S. 1998. Clinical Review 94: What's in a Name? In Search of Leptin's Physiologic Role. *Journal of Clinical Endocrinology and Metabolism* 83:1407–13.

Flier, J. S. 2004. Obesity Wars: Molecular Progress Confronts an Expanding Epidemic. *Cell* 116:337–50.

Flier, J. S., M. Harris, and A. N. Hollenberg. 2000. Leptin, Nutrition, and the Thyroid: The Why, the Wherefore, and the Wiring. *Journal of Clinical Investigation* 105:859–61.

Fonseca, V., S. Dejager, D. Albrecht, L. Shirt, and A. Schweizer. 2006. Galvus as Add-on to Insulin in Patients with Type 2 Diabetes (T2DM). Paper presented at the meeting of the American Diabetes Association, Washington, DC.

Friedman, J. M., and J. L. Halaas. 1998. Leptin and the Regulation of Body Weight in Mammals. *Nature* 395:763–70.

Fruhbeck, G., J. Gomez-Ambrosi, F. J. Muruzabal, and M. A. Burrell. 2001. The Adipocyte: A Model for Integration of Endocrine and Metabolic Signaling in Energy Metabolism Regulation. *American Journal of Physiology, Endocrinology and Metabolism* 280:E827–47.

Fukuhara, A., M. Matsuda, M. Nishizawa, K. Segawa, M. Tanaka, K. Kishimoto, Y. Matsuki, et al. 2005. Visfatin: A Protein Secreted by Visceral Fat That Mimics the Effects of Insulin. *Science* 307:426–30.

Gannage-Yared, M. H., S. Khalife, M. Semaan, F. Fares, S. Jambart, and G. Halaby. 2006. Serum Adiponectin and Leptin Levels in Relation to the Metabolic Syndrome, Androgenic Profile and Somatotropic Axis in Healthy Non-Diabetic Elderly Men. *European Journal of Endocrinology* 155:167–76.

Ginsberg, H. N., Y. L. Zhang, and A. Hernandez-Ono. 2006. Metabolic Syndrome: Focus on Dyslipidemia. *Obesity* 14. Suppl. no.1. 41S–49S.

Gorden, P., and O. Gavrilova. 2003. The Clinical Uses of Leptin. *Current Opinion in Pharmacology* 3:655–59.

Grujic, D., V. S. Susulic, M. E. Harper, J. Himms-Hagen, B. A. Cunningham, B. E. Corkey, and B. B. Lowell. 1997. Beta3-adrenergic Receptors on White and Brown Adipocytes Mediate Beta3-selective Agonist-Induced Effects on Energy Expenditure, Insulin Secretion, and Food Intake. *Journal of Biological Chemistry* 272:17686–93.

Halaas, J. L., K. S. Gajiwala, M. Maffei, et al. 1995. Weight-Reducing Effects of the Plasma Protein Encoded by the Obese Gene. *Science Magazine* 269:543–546.

Halperin, F., J. A. Beckman, M. E. Patti, M. E. Trujillo, M. Garvin, M. A. Creager, P. E. Scherer, and A. B. Goldfine. 2005. The Role of Total and High-Molecular-Weight Complex of Adiponectin in Vascular Function in Offspring Whose Parents Both Had Type 2 Diabetes. *Diabetologia* 48:2147–54.

Hara, K., P. Boutin, Y. Mori, K. Tobe, C. Dina, K. Yasuda, T. Yamauchi, et al. 2002. Genetic Variation in the Gene Encoding Adiponectin is Associated with an Increased Risk of Type 2 Diabetes in the Japanese Population. *Diabetes* 51:536–40.

Henson M. C., and V. D. Castracane. 2006. Leptin in Pregnancy: An Update. *Biology of Reproduction* 74:218–29.

Hileman, S. M., D. D. Pierroz, and J. S. Flier. 2000. Leptin, Nutrition, and Reproduction: Timing Is Everything. *Journal of Clinical Endocrinology and Metabolism* 85:804–807.

Hotamisligil, G. S., N. S. Shargill, and B. M. Spiegelman. 1993. Adipose Expression of Tumor Necrosis Factor: Direct Tole in Obesity-Linked Insulin Resistance. *Science Magazine* 259:87–91.

Hotta, K., T. Funahashi, N. L. Bodkin, H. K. Ortmeyer, Y. Arita, B. C. Hansen, and Y. Matsuzawa. 2001. Circulating Concentrations of the Adipocyte Protein Adiponectin Are Decreased in Parallel with Reduced Insulin Sensitivity During the Progression to Type 2 Diabetes in Rhesus Monkeys. *Diabetes* 50:1126–33.

Hu, E., P. Liang, and B. M. Spiegelman. 1996. AdipoQ is a Novel Adipose-Specific Gene Dysregulated in Obesity. *Journal of Biological Chemistry* 271:10697–703.

Ionsidine, R. V., M. K. Sinha, M. L. Heiman, et al. 1996. Serum Immunoreactive Leptin Concentrations in Normal-weight and Obese Humans. *New England Journal of Medicine* 334:292–95.

Isganaitis, E., and R. H. Lustig. 2005. Fast Food, Central Nervous System Insulin Resistance, and Obesity. *Arteriosclerosis, Thrombosis, and Vascular Biology* 25:2451.

Iyengar, P., T. P. Combs, S. J. Shah, V. Gouon-Evans, J. W. Pollard, C. Albanese, L. Flanagan, et al. 2003. Adipocyte Secreted Factors Synergistically Promote Mammary Tumorigenesis Through Induction of Anti-Apoptotic Transcriptional Programs and Proto-oncogene Stabilization. *Oncogene* 22:6408–23.

Iyengar, P., V. Espina, T. W. Williams, Y. Lin, D. Berry, L. A. Jelicks, H. Lee, et al. 2005. Adipocyte-Derived Collagen VI Affects Early Mammary Tumor Progression in Vivo, Demonstrating a Critical Interaction in the Tumor/stroma Microenvironment. *Journal of Clinical Investigation* 115:1163–76.

Kantartzis, K., A. Fritsche, O. Tschritter, C. Thamer, M. Haap, S. Schafer, M. Stumvoll, H. U. Haring, and N. Stefan. 2005. The

Association Between Plasma Adiponectin and Insulin Sensitivity in Humans Depends on Obesity. *Obesity* 13:1683–91.

Kim, S. G., O. H. Ryu, H. Y. Kim, K. W. Lee, J. A Seo, N. H. Kim, K. M. Choi, J. Lee, S. H. Baik, and D. S. Choi. 2006. Effect of Rosiglitazone on Plasma Adiponectin Levels and Arterial Stiffness in Subjects with Prediabetes or Non-Diabetic Metabolic Syndrome. *European Journal of Endocrinology* 154:433–40.

Kubota, N., Y. Terauchi, T. Yamauchi, T. Kubota, M. Moroi, J. Matsui, K. Eto, et al. 2002. Disruption of Adiponectin Causes Insulin Resistance and Neointimal Formation. *Journal of Biological Chemistry* 277:25863–66.

Kubota, N. Y., T. Terauchi, H. Kubota, S. Kumagai, H. Itoh, W. Satoh, H. Yano, et al. 2006. Pioglitazone Ameliorates Insulin Resistance and Diabetes by Both Adiponectin-Dependent and -Independent Pathways. *Journal of Biological Chemistry* 281:8748–55.

Laposky, A. D., J. Shelton, J. Bass, C. Dugovic, N. Perrino, and F. W. Turek. 2006. Altered Sleep Regulation in Leptin-Deficient Mice. *American Journal of Physiology: Regulatory, Integrative and Comparative Physiology* 290:R894–903.

Lara-Castro, C., N. Luo, P. Wallace, R. L. Klein, and W. T. Garvey. 2006. Adiponectin Multimeric Complexes and the Metabolic Syndrome Trait Cluster. *Diabetes* 55:249–259.

Lazar, M. A. 2005. How Obesity Causes Diabetes: Not a Tall Tale. *Science Magazine* 307:373–75.

Lee, G. H., R. Proenca, J. M. Montez, K. M. Carroll, J.G. Darvishzadeh, J. I. Lee, and J. M. Friedman. 1996. Abnormal Splicing of the Leptin Receptor in Diabetic Mice. *Nature* 379:632–35.

Lin, Y., A. H. Berg, P. Iyengar, T. K. Lam, A. Giacca, T. P. Combs, M. W. Rajala, et al. 2005. The Hyperglycemia-Induced Inflammatory Response in Adipocytes: The Role of Reactive Oxygen Species. *Journal of Biological Chemistry* 280:4617–26.

Lin, Y., M. W. Rajala, J. P. Berger, D. E. Moller, N. Barzilai, and P. E. Scherer. 2001. Hyperglycemia-Induced Production of Acute Phase Reactants in Adipose Tissue. *Journal of Biological Chemistry* 276:42077–83.

Linnquist, F., P. Arner, L. Nordfors, et al. 1995. Overexpression of the Obese (ob) Gene in Adipose Tissue of Human Obese Subjects. *Nature Medicine* 1:950–53.

Maeda, K., K. Okubo, I. Shimomura, T. Funahashi, Y. Matsuzawa, and K. Matsubara. 1996. cDNA Cloning and Expression of a Novel Adipose Specific Collagen-like Factor, apM1 (AdiPose Most abundant Gene transcript 1). *Biochemistry and Biophysics Research Communications* 221:286-89.

Maeda, K., K. Okubo, I. Shimomura, K. Mizuno, Y. Matsuzawa, and K. Matsubara. 1997. Analysis of an Expression Profile of Genes in the Human Adipose Tissue. *Gene* 190:227–35.

Maeda, N., I. Shimomura, K. Kishida, H. Nishizawa, M. Matsuda, H. Nagaretani, N. Furuyama, et al. 2002. Diet-Induced Insulin Resistance in Mice Lacking Adiponectin/ACRP30. *Nature Medicine* 8:731–37.

Maffei, M., J. Halaas, E. Ravussin, et al. 1995. Leptin Levels in Human and Rodent: Measurement of Plasma Leptin and ob RNA in Obese and Weight-Reduced Subjects. *Nature Medicine* 1:1155-61.

Margetic, S., C. Gazzola, G. G. Pegg, and R.A. Hill. 2002. Leptin: A Review of Its Peripheral Actions and Interactions. *International Journal of Obesity and Related Metabolic Disorders* 26:1407–33.

Masuzaki, H., Y. Ogawa, N. Isse, et al. 1995. Human Obese Gene Expression: Adipocyte-Specific Expression and Regional Differences in the Adipose Tissue. *Diabetes* 44:855-58.

Masuzaki, H., J. Paterson, H. Shinyama, N. M. Morton, J. J. Mullins, J. R. Seckl, and J. S. Flier. 2001. A Transgenic Model of Visceral Obesity and the Metabolic Syndrome. *Science* 294:2166–70.

Meseguer, A., C. Puche, and A. Cabero. 2002. Sex Steroid Biosynthesis in White Adipose Tissue. *Hormone and Metabolic Research* 34:731–36.

Moitra, J., M. M. Mason, M. Olive, D. Krylov, O. Gavrilova, B. Marcus-Samuels, L. Feigenbaum, et al. 1998. Life Without White Fat: A Transgenic Mouse. *Genes and Development* 12:3168-81.

Nakano, Y., T. Tobe, N. H. Choi-Miura, T. Mazda, and M. Tomita. 1996. Isolation and Characterization of GBP28, a Novel Gelatin-Binding Protein Purified From Human Plasma. *Journal of Biochemistry* (Tokyo) 120:803-12.

Nawrocki, A. R., M. W. Rajala, E. Tomas, U. B. Pajvani, A. K. Saha, M. E. Trumbauer, Z. Pang, et al. 2006. Mice Lacking Adiponectin Show Decreased Hepatic Insulin Sensitivity and Reduced Responsiveness to Peroxisome Proliferator-Activated Receptor Gamma Agonists. *Journal of Biological Chemistry* 281:2654-60.

Nawrocki, A. R., and P. E. Scherer. 2005. Keynote Review: The Adipocyte as a Drug Discovery Target. *Drug Discovery Today* 10:1219-30.

Otto, T. C., and M. D. Lane. 2005. Adipose Development: From Stem Cell to Adipocyte. *Critical Reviews in Biochemistry and Molecular Biology* 40:229–42.

Pajvani, U. B., X. Du, T. P. Combs, A. H. Berg, M. W. Rajala, T. Schulthess, J. Engel, M. Brownlee, and P. E. Scherer. 2003. Structure-function Studies of the Adipocyte-Secreted Hormone Acrp30/adiponectin: Implications for Metabolic Regulation and Bioactivity. *Journal of Biological Chemistry* 278:9073-85.

Pajvani, U. B., M. Hawkins, T. P. Combs, M. W. Rajala, T. Doebber, J. P. Berger, J. A. Wagner, et al. 2004. Complex Distribution, Not Absolute Amount of Adiponectin, Correlates with

Thiazolidinedione: Mediated Improvement in Insulin Sensitivity. *Journal of Biological Chemistry* 279:12152-62.

Pajvani, U. B., M. E. Trujillo, T. P. Combs, P. Iyengar, L. Jelicks, K. A. Roth, R. N. Kitsis, and P. E. Scherer. 2005. Fat Apoptosis Through Targeted Activation of Caspase 8: A New Mouse Model of Inducible and Reversible Lipoatrophy. *Nature Medicine* 11:797-803.

Patel, S. D., M. W. Rajala, L. Rossetti, P. E. Scherer, and L. Shapiro. 2004. Disulfide-Dependent Multimeric Assembly of Resistin Family Hormones. *Science Magazine* 304:1154-58.

Pelleymounter, M. A., M. J. Cullen, M. B. Baker, et al. 1995. Effects of the Obese Gene Product on Body Weight Regulation in ob/ob Mice. *Science Magazine* 269:540-43.

Raben, A., T. Vasilaras, C. Moiler, and A. Astrup. 2002. Sucrose Compared with Artificial Sweeteners: Different Effects on ad Libitum Food Intake and Body Weight After 10 wk of Supplementation in Overweight Subjects. *American Journal of Clinical Nutrition* 76(4):721–29 [Correspondence: A. Raben. Research Dept of Human Nutrition, Centre for Advanced Food Studies, The Royal Veterinary & Agricultural University, 30 Roligheclsvej, DK-1958 Frederiksberg C, Denmark.]

Rajala, M. W., Y. Lin, M. Ranalletta, X. M. Yang, H. Qian, R. Gingerich, N. Barzilai, and P. E. Scherer. 2002. Cell Type-Specific Expression and Coregulation of Murine Resistin and Resistin-like Molecule-alpha in Adipose Tissue. *Molecular Endocrinology* 16:1920-30.

Rajala, M. W., S. Obici, P. E. Scherer, and L. Rossetti. 2003. Adipose-Derived Resistin and Gut-Derived Resistin-like Molecule-ß Selectively Impair Insulin Action on Glucose Production. *Journal of Clinical Investigation* 111:225–30.

Rosenstock, J., M. Baron, A. Schweizer, D. Mills, and S. Dejager. 2006. Galvus Is as Effective as Rosiglitazone in Lowering HbA1c but without Weight Gain in Drug-Naive Patients with

Type 2 Diabetes (T2DM). Paper presented at the meeting of the American Diabetes Association, Washington, DC.

Ross, S. R., R. A. Graves, and B. M. Spiegelman. 1993. Targeted Expression of a Toxin Gene to Adipose Tissue: Transgenic Mice Resistant to Obesity. *Genes and Development* 7:1318–24.

Roth, J. 2006. Leptin Responsivity Restored in Leptin-Resistant Diet-Induced Obese (DIO) Rats: Synergistic Actions of Amylin and Leptin for Reduction in Body Weight (BW) and Fat. Poster presented at the American Diabetes Association Poster Session.

Rothenbacher, D., H. Brenner, W. Marz, and W. Koenig. 2005. Adiponectin, Risk of Coronary Heart Disease and Correlations with Cardiovascular Risk Markers. *European Heart Journal* 26:1640–46.

Salmenniemi, U., J. Zacharova, E. Ruotsalainen, I. Vauhkonen, J. Pihlajamaki, S. Kainulainen, K. Punnonen, and M. Laakso. 2005. Association of Adiponectin Level and Variants in the Adiponectin Gene with Glucose Metabolism, Energy Expenditure, and Cytokines in Offspring of Type 2 Diabetic Patients. *Journal of Clinical Endocrinology and Metabolism* 90:4216–23.

Saydah, S. H., J. Fradkin, and C. C. Cowie. 2004. Poor Control of Risk Factors for Vascular Disease Among Adults with Previously Diagnosed Diabetes. *Journal of the American Medical Association* 291:335–42.

Scherer, P. E., S. Williams, M. Fogliano, G. Baldini, and H. F. Lodish. 1995. A Novel Serum Protein Similar to C1q, Produced Exclusively in Adipocytes. *Journal of Biological Chemistry* 270:26746–49.

Shimomura, I., R. E. Hammer, J. A. Richardson, S. Ikemoto, Y. Bashmakov, J. L. Goldstein, and M. S. Brown. 1998. Insulin Resistance and Diabetes Mellitus in Transgenic Mice Expressing Nuclear SREBP-1c in Adipose Tissue: Model for

Congenital Generalized Lipodystrophy. *Genes and Development* 12:3182–94.

Siiteri, P. K. 1987. Adipose Tissue as a Source of Hormones. *American Journal of Clinical Nutrition* 45:277–82.

Steppan, C. M., S. T. Bailey, S. Bhat, E. J. Brown, R. R. Banerjee, C. M. Wright, H. R. Patel, R. S. Ahima, and M. A. Lazar. 2001. The Hormone Resistin Links Obesity to Diabetes. *Nature* 409:307–12.

Steppan, C. M., E. J. Brown, C. M. Wright, S. Bhat, R. R. Banerjee, C. Y. Dai, G. H. Enders, D. G. Silberg, X. Wen, G. D. Wu, and M. A. Lazar. 2001. A Family of Tissue-Specific Resistin-like Molecules. *Proceedings of the National Academy of Sciences of the U.S.A.* 98:502-26.

Stumvoll, M., O. Tschritter, A. Fritsche, H. Staiger, W. Renn, M. Weisser, F. Machicao, and H. Haring. 2002. Association of the T-G Polymorphism in Adiponectin (exon 2) with Obesity and Insulin Sensitivity: Interaction with Family History of Type 2 Diabetes. *Diabetes* 51:37–41.

Tartaglia, L. A., M. Dembski, X. Weng, N. Deng, J. Culpepper, R. Devos, G. J. Richards, L. A. Campfield, F. T. Clark, J. Deeds, et al. 1995. Identification and Expression Cloning of a Leptin Receptor, OB-R. *Cell* 83:1263–71.

Umpierrez, G. E., S. D. Isaacs, N. Bazargan, X. You, L. M. Thaler, and A. E. Kitabchi. 2002. Hyperglycemia: An Independent Marker of In-hospital Mortality Among Hospitalized Patients. *Journal of Clinical Endocrinology and Metabolism* 87:978–82.

Wajchenberg, B. L. 2000. Subcutaneous and Visceral Adipose Tissue: Their Relation to the Metabolic Syndrome. *Endocrinolgy Review* 21:697–738.

Wang, A. Y., I. J. Hickman, A. A. Richards, J. P. Whitehead, J. B. Prins, and G. A. Macdonald. 2005. High Molecular Weight Adiponectin Correlates with Insulin Sensitivity in Patients with

Hepatitis C Genotype 3, but not Genotype 1 Infection. *American Journal of Gastroenterology* 100:2717–23.

Weisberg, S. P., D. McCann, M. Desai, M. Rosenbaum, R. L. Leibel, and A. W. Ferrante Jr. 2003. Obesity Is Associated with Macrophage Accumulation in Adipose Tissue. *Journal of Clinical Investigation* 112:1796–1808.

Wellen, K. E., and G. S. Hotamisligil. 2003. Obesity-Induced Inflammatory Changes in Adipose Tissue. *Journal of Clinical Investigation* 112:1785–88.

Xu, H., G. T. Barnes, Q. Yang, G. Tan, D. Yang, C. J. Chou, J. Sole, A. Nichols, J. S. Ross, L. A. Tartaglia, and H. Chen. 2003. Chronic Inflammation in Fat Plays a Crucial Role in the Development of Obesity-Related Insulin Resistance. *Journal of Clinical Investigation* 112:1821–30.

Yamauchi, T., J. Kamon, Y. Ito, A. Tsuchida, T. Yokomizo, S. Kita, T. Sugiyama, et al. 2003. Cloning of Adiponectin Receptors that Mediate Antidiabetic Metabolic Effects. *Nature* 423:762–69.

Yang, Q., T. E. Graham, N. Mody, F. Preitner, O. D. Peroni, J. M. Zabolotny, K. Kotani, L. Quadro, and B. B. Kahn. 2005. Serum Retinol Binding Protein 4 Contributes to Insulin Resistance in Obesity and Type 2 Diabetes. *Nature* 436:356–62.

Zhang, Y., R. Proenca, M. Maffel, M. Barone, L. Leopold, and J. M. Friedman. 1994. Positional Cloning of the Mouse Obese Gene and its Human Homologue. *Nature* 372:425–32.

INDEX

About the Author

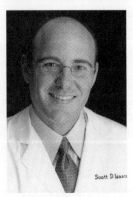

Scott D Isaac

Scott Isaacs, M.D., F.A.C.P., F.A.C.E., is a board-certified endocrinologist in Atlanta, Georgia, where he is the medical director at Intelligent Health Center, a multidisciplinary center for the treatment of endocrine disorders and obesity. He conducts research on obesity, stress, and diabetes and has published many articles in peer-reviewed medical journals, including the *Journal of Endocrinology and Metabolism, Diabetes Care* and the *Journal of Critical Care.*

Dr. Isaacs is also a clinical instructor of medicine at Emory University School of Medicine. He attended Emory School of Medicine and continued on at Emory for his residency and fellowship in endocrinology, diabetes, and metabolism. He gives many lectures on the subject of hormones and obesity, speaking to groups in the community as well as at major events and conferences throughout the United States. He also trains other doctors in the field.

Dr. Isaacs has been quoted in many national publications and websites, including *Better Homes and Gardens, Better Health and Living, Women's Health and Fitness, Prevention, Real Simple, The Atlanta Journal-Constitution, The Chicago Tribune, Men's Health, Fitness Magazine, Glamour, Alternative Medicine, Women's World, First Health, WebMD,* and many others. He has also given expert commentary on several radio and television news programs.

Author of *Hormonal Balance: Understanding Hormones, Weight, and Your Metabolism* (Bull Publishing), *A Simple Guide to Thyroid Disorders: From Diagnosis to Treatment* (Addicus Books), and *Overcoming Metabolic Syndrome* (Addicus Books), Dr. Isaacs is also an officer of the Georgia chapter of the American Association of Clinical Endocrinologists and is the medical advisor for Cushing's Understanding, Support, and Help Organization. Furthermore, Dr. Isaacs is a Diplomat of the American Board of Bariatric Medicine, a Fellow of the American College of Physicians (FACP), and a Fellow of the American College of Clinical Endocrinology (FACE). He may be reached through his website: *www.IntelligentHealthCenter.com.*